Newborn Screening for Sickle Cell Disease and other Haemoglobinopathies

Newborn Screening for Sickle Cell Disease and other Haemoglobinopathies

Special Issue Editors

Stephan Lobitz
Jacques Elion
Raffaella Colombatti
Elena Cela

MDPI • Basel • Beijing • Wuhan • Barcelona • Belgrade

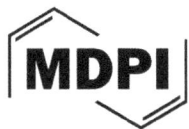

Special Issue Editors

Stephan Lobitz
Gemeinschaftsklinikum Mittelrhein gGmbH
Germany

Jacques Elion
Université Paris Diderot-USPC
France

Raffaella Colombatti
Università di Padova
Italy

Elena Cela
Universidad Complutense de Madrid
Spain

Editorial Office
MDPI
St. Alban-Anlage 66
4052 Basel, Switzerland

This is a reprint of articles from the Special Issue published online in the open access journal *International Journal of Neonatal Screening* (ISSN 2409-515X) from 2018 to 2019 (available at: https://www.mdpi.com/journal/IJNS/special_issues/hemoglobinopathies)

For citation purposes, cite each article independently as indicated on the article page online and as indicated below:

LastName, A.A.; LastName, B.B.; LastName, C.C. Article Title. *Journal Name* **Year**, *Article Number*, Page Range.

ISBN 978-3-03921-614-7 (Pbk)
ISBN 978-3-03921-615-4 (PDF)

© 2019 by the authors. Articles in this book are Open Access and distributed under the Creative Commons Attribution (CC BY) license, which allows users to download, copy and build upon published articles, as long as the author and publisher are properly credited, which ensures maximum dissemination and a wider impact of our publications.

The book as a whole is distributed by MDPI under the terms and conditions of the Creative Commons license CC BY-NC-ND.

Contents

About the Special Issue Editors vii

Raffaella Colombatti, Elena Cela, Jacques Elion and Stephan Lobitz
Editorial for Special Issue "Newborn Screening for Sickle Cell Disease and other Haemoglobinopathies"
Reprinted from: *Int. J. Neonatal Screen.* **2019**, *5*, 36, doi:10.3390/ijns5040036 . . . . **1**

J. Gerard Loeber
European Union Should Actively Stimulate and Harmonise Neonatal Screening Initiatives
Reprinted from: *Int. J. Neonatal Screen.* **2018**, *4*, 32, doi:10.3390/ijns4040032 . . . . **3**

Baba P.D. Inusa, Lewis L. Hsu, Neeraj Kohli, Anissa Patel, Kilali Ominu-Evbota, Kofi A. Anie and Wale Atoyebi
Sickle Cell Disease—Genetics, Pathophysiology, Clinical Presentation and Treatment
Reprinted from: *Int. J. Neonatal Screen.* **2019**, *5*, 20, doi:10.3390/ijns5020020 . . . . **8**

Michael Angastiniotis and Stephan Lobitz
Thalassemias: An Overview
Reprinted from: *Int. J. Neonatal Screen.* **2019**, *5*, 16, doi:10.3390/ijns5010016 . . . . **23**

Claudia Frömmel
Newborn Screening for Sickle Cell Disease and Other Hemoglobinopathies: A Short Review on Classical Laboratory Methods—Isoelectric Focusing, HPLC, and Capillary Electrophoresis
Reprinted from: *Int. J. Neonatal Screen.* **2018**, *4*, 39, doi:10.3390/ijns4040039 . . . . **34**

Yvonne Daniel and Charles Turner
Newborn Sickle Cell Disease Screening Using Electrospray Tandem Mass Spectrometry
Reprinted from: *Int. J. Neonatal Screen.* **2018**, *4*, 35, doi:10.3390/ijns4040035 . . . . **44**

Pierre Naubourg, Marven El Osta, David Rageot, Olivier Grunewald, Gilles Renom, Patrick Ducoroy and Jean-Marc Périni
A Multicentre Pilot Study of a Two-Tier Newborn Sickle Cell Disease Screening Procedure with a First Tier Based on a Fully Automated MALDI-TOF MS Platform
Reprinted from: *Int. J. Neonatal Screen.* **2019**, *5*, 10, doi:10.3390/ijns5010010 . . . . **49**

Maddalena Martella, Giampietro Viola, Silvia Azzena, Sara Schiavon, Andrea Biondi, Giuseppe Basso, Paola Corti, Raffaella Colombatti, Nicoletta Masera and Laura Sainati
Evaluation of Technical Issues in a Pilot Multicenter Newborn Screening Program for Sickle Cell Disease
Reprinted from: *Int. J. Neonatal Screen.* **2019**, *5*, 2, doi:10.3390/ijns5010002 . . . . **62**

Yvonne Daniel, Jacques Elion, Bichr Allaf, Catherine Badens, Marelle J. Bouva, Ian Brincat, Elena Cela, Cathy Coppinger, Mariane de Montalembert, Béatrice Gulbis, Joan Henthorn, Olivier Ketelslegers, Corrina McMahon, Allison Streetly, Raffaella Colombatti and Stephan Lobitz
Newborn Screening for Sickle Cell Disease in Europe
Reprinted from: *Int. J. Neonatal Screen.* **2019**, *5*, 15, doi:10.3390/ijns5010015 . . . . **70**

Béatrice Gulbis, Phu-Quoc Lê, Olivier Ketelslegers, Marie-Françoise Dresse, Anne-Sophie Adam, Frédéric Cotton, François Boemer, Vincent Bours, Jean-Marc Minon and Alina Ferster
Neonatal Screening for Sickle Cell Disease in Belgium for More than 20 Years: An Experience for Comprehensive Care Improvement
Reprinted from: *Int. J. Neonatal Screen.* **2018**, *4*, 37, doi:10.3390/ijns4040037 82

Nura El-Haj and Carolyn C. Hoppe
Newborn Screening for SCD in the USA and Canada
Reprinted from: *Int. J. Neonatal Screen.* **2018**, *4*, 36, doi:10.3390/ijns4040036 90

Jennifer Knight-Madden, Ketty Lee, Gisèle Elana, Narcisse Elenga, Beatriz Marcheco-Teruel, Ngozi Keshi, Maryse Etienne-Julan, Lesley King, Monika Asnani, Marc Romana and Marie-Dominique Hardy-Dessources
Newborn Screening for Sickle Cell Disease in the Caribbean: An Update of the Present Situation and of the Disease Prevalence
Reprinted from: *Int. J. Neonatal Screen.* **2019**, *5*, 5, doi:10.3390/ijns5010005 100

Ana C. Silva-Pinto, Maria Cândida Alencar de Queiroz, Paula Juliana Antoniazzo Zamaro, Miranete Arruda and Helena Pimentel dos Santos
The Neonatal Screening Program in Brazil, Focus on Sickle Cell Disease (SCD)
Reprinted from: *Int. J. Neonatal Screen.* **2019**, *5*, 11, doi:10.3390/ijns5010011 109

Roshan B. Colah, Pallavi Mehta and Malay B. Mukherjee
Newborn Screening for Sickle Cell Disease: Indian Experience
Reprinted from: *Int. J. Neonatal Screen.* **2018**, *4*, 31, doi:10.3390/ijns4040031 116

Athena Anderle, Germana Bancone, Gonzalo J. Domingo, Emily Gerth-Guyette, Sampa Pal and Ari W. Satyagraha
Point-of-Care Testing for G6PD Deficiency: Opportunities for Screening
Reprinted from: *Int. J. Neonatal Screen.* **2018**, *4*, 34, doi:10.3390/ijns4040034 124

John James and Elizabeth Dormandy
Improving Screening Programmes for Sickle Cell Disorders and Other Haemoglobinopathies in Europe: The Role of Patient Organisations
Reprinted from: *Int. J. Neonatal Screen.* **2019**, *5*, 12, doi:10.3390/ijns5010012 137

Baba P.D. Inusa, Kofi A. Anie, Andrea Lamont, Livingstone G. Dogara, Bola Ojo, Ifeoma Ijei, Wale Atoyebi, Larai Gwani, Esther Gani and Lewis Hsu
Utilising the 'Getting to Outcomes®' Framework in Community Engagement for Development and Implementation of Sickle Cell Disease Newborn Screening in Kaduna State, Nigeria
Reprinted from: *Int. J. Neonatal Screen.* **2018**, *4*, 33, doi:10.3390/ijns4040033 141

About the Special Issue Editors

Stephan Lobitz is the director of the Department of Pediatric Hematology and Oncology at Gemeinschaftsklinikum Mittelrhein in Koblenz, Germany. He studied Medicine and Hemoglobinopathies in Düsseldorf, Berlin, and London, and trained at Charité University Hospital in Berlin. He is the spokesperson of the Sickle Cell Disease Management Program of the German Society of Pediatric Hematology and Oncology and the coordinator of the German Sickle Cell Disease Treatment Guideline. Dr. Lobitz has a special interest in newborn screening and coordinated the recent European consensus statement on newborn screening for sickle cell disease.

Jacques Elion received his MD from Paris Descartes and a PhD from Paris Diderot Universities. He was a Research Assistant at the Mayo Graduate School of Medicine, University of Minnesota and a Fogarty Scientist at the US National Institutes of Health. Dr Elion is Professor of Molecular Genetics at the Université de Paris and Visiting Professor at the Universidade de São Paulo. He is the former Director of the Dept of Medical Genetics at the Robert Debré University Hospital. Dr Elion's research is focused on the pathophysiology, prevention, and global care of SCD. It is conducted at Unit 1134 of the French National Institute of Health and Medical Research (Inserm) sheltered by the National Institute of Blood Transfusion in Paris and at the University Hospital in Guadeloupe. The Unit is part of the French Laboratory of Excellence on the Red Cell (GR-Ex). Dr Elion has developed extensive international collaborations, notably in sub-Saharan Africa, India, the Caribbean, and Brazil. Dr Elion has organized and chaired several international meetings, including the scientific session at the inaugural ceremony for the 1st World SCD Day, 19 June 2009, UN Headquarters, NYC.

Raffaella Colombatti is a pediatric hematologist and oncologist at Padova University in Italy. She is the coordinator of the Red Cell Disorder Working Group of the Italian Association of Pediatric Hematology Oncology (AIEOP) and the Vice Chair of the Veneto Region Reference Center for the Diagnosis and Treatment of Sickle Cell Disease in Childhood and the Pilot Universal Newborn Screening Program for Sickle Cell Disease. Her main interests are in hemoglobinopathies and child global health care.

Elena Cela graduated at Complutense University in Madrid, Spain and specialized in pediatric hematology and oncology. She is the coordinator of the hemoglobinopathy group of the Spanish Society of Pediatric Hematology and Oncology (SEHOP) and the Spanish Registry of Hemoglobinopathies (REHem). Prof. Cela is the head of the Department of Pediatric Hematology and Oncology at Hospital Gregorio Marañón in Madrid, which is a referral center for erythropathology. She contributed to the implementation of the Spanish newborn screening for sickle cell disease in Madrid in 2003 and coordinated the edition of the Spanish guidelines on sickle cell disease (2010 and 2019). Her main interests are red cell disorders and newborn screening.

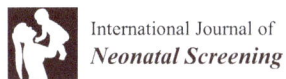

Editorial

Editorial for Special Issue "Newborn Screening for Sickle Cell Disease and other Haemoglobinopathies"

Raffaella Colombatti [1,*], Elena Cela [2], Jacques Elion [3] and Stephan Lobitz [4]

1. Department of Child and Maternal Health, Clinic of Pediatric Hematology/Oncology, Azienda Ospedaliera-Università di Padova, 35129 Padova, Italy
2. Department of Pediatric Oncology/Hematology, Hospital Universitario General Gregorio Marañón, Facultad de Medicina, Universidad Complutense Madrid, 28007 Madrid, Spain; elena.cela@salud.madrid.org
3. Laboratoire d'Excellence GR-Ex, UMR_S1134, Inserm, Université Paris Diderot, Sorbonne Paris Cité, Institut National de la Transfusion Sanguine, 75015 Paris, France; jacques.elion@inserm.fr
4. Department of Pediatric Hematology and Oncology, Gemeinschaftsklinikum Mittelrhein gGmbH, 56073 Koblenz, Germany; Stephan.Lobitz@gk.de
* Correspondence: rcolombatti@gmail.com

Received: 17 September 2019; Accepted: 17 September 2019; Published: 20 September 2019

Sickle cell disease (SCD) is among the most common genetic disorders in the world, affecting over 300,000 newborns annually, with estimates for further increases to over 400,000 annual births within the next generation and with a wider geographical distribution of affected individuals due to global migration [1,2]. Both the World Health Organization (WHO) and the United Nations have identified SCD as a current global health burden [3,4].

The optimal care for children with SCD starts with newborn screening (NBS), which can establish a diagnosis before the onset of symptoms and allow early interventions such as prophylactic penicillin, pneumococcal immunization, screening with Transcranial Doppler ultrasound, caregiver education, and comprehensive care [5]. NBS followed by adequate comprehensive care reduce morbidity, mortality, and healthcare costs while improving the quality of life for patients.

Universal NBS is now recommended in the United States, Europe, and Brazil, although widespread implementation still needs to be achieved and many challenges remain to ensure that every child with SCD is diagnosed through NBS [6,7].

In this Special Issue on Newborn Screening for Sickle Cell Disease and Other Hemoglobinopathies (https://www.mdpi.com/journal/IJNS/special_issues/hemoglobinopathies), we have assembled a collection of review and original articles.

We have tried to cover the most widely faced challenges in the field of newborn screening for SCD: unmet needs in Europe and healthcare policy implementation as well as patient involvement and development of new diagnostic techniques.

We would like to commend the authors for the excellent reviews on the pathophysiology of SCD and thalassemia, the state of the art of NBS at a global level, and the technologies available for NBS. We would also like to praise the authors who provided original articles on specific technical topics which understanding is essential for more reliable, technically sound, and faster diagnosis.

Global diseases can be tackled only with global and coordinated efforts of different experts ranging from clinicians to technicians and basic scientists, as well as healthcare planners and the patients themselves across different countries. This Special Issue brings together a multidisciplinary global team presenting the actual situation and proposals for future developments.

Conflicts of Interest: The authors declare no conflict of interest.

References

1. Piel, F.B.; Tatem, A.J.; Huang, Z.; Gupta, S.; Williams, T.N.; Weatherall, D.J. Global migration and the changing distribution of sickle haemoglobin: A quantitative study of temporal trends between 1960 and 2000. *Lancet Glob. Health* **2014**, *2*, e80–e89. [CrossRef]
2. Piel, F.B.; Hay, S.I.; Gupta, S.; Weatherall, D.J.; Williams, T.N. Global burden of sickle cell anaemia in children under five, 2010–2050: Modelling based on demographics, excess mortality, and interventions. *PLoS Med.* **2013**, *10*, e1001484. [CrossRef] [PubMed]
3. WHO Report A59/9 on Sickle Cell Anemia. 2006. Available online: www.who.int/gb/ebwha/pdf_files/WHA59-REC1/e/WHA59_2006_REC1-en.pdf (accessed on 18 September 2019).
4. UN Resolution A/63/L.63 "Recognition of Sickle-Cell Anaemia as a Public Health Problem". 2008. Available online: www.un.org/News/Press/docs/2008/ga10803.doc.htm (accessed on 18 Sepember 2019).
5. Yawn, B.P.; Buchanan, G.R.; Afenyi-Annan, A.N.; Ballas, S.K.; Hassell, K.L.; James, A.H.; Jordan, L.; Lanzkron, S.M.; Lottenberg, R.; Savage, W.J.; et al. Management of sickle cell disease: Summary of the 2014 evidence-based report by expert panel members. *JAMA* **2014**, *312*, 1033–1048. [CrossRef] [PubMed]
6. Shook, L.M.; Ware, R.E. Sickle cell screening in Europe: The time has come. *Br. J. Haematol.* **2018**, *183*, 534–535. [CrossRef] [PubMed]
7. Lobitz, S.; Telfer, P.; Cela, E.; Allaf, B.; Angastiniotis, M.; Backman Johansson, C.; Badens, C.; Bento, C.; Bouva, M.J.; Canatan, D.; et al. Newborn screening for sickle cell disease in Europe: recommendations from a Pan-European Consensus Conference. *Br. J. Haematol.* **2018**, *183*, 648–660. [CrossRef] [PubMed]

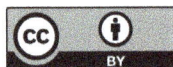

© 2019 by the authors. Licensee MDPI, Basel, Switzerland. This article is an open access article distributed under the terms and conditions of the Creative Commons Attribution (CC BY) license (http://creativecommons.org/licenses/by/4.0/).

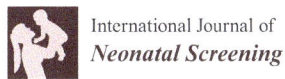

Editorial

European Union Should Actively Stimulate and Harmonise Neonatal Screening Initiatives

J. Gerard Loeber

International Society for Neonatal Screening Office, Burgemeester Fabiuspark 55, 3721CK Bilthoven, The Netherlands; gerard.loeber@gmail.com; Tel.: +31-6-4616-3922

Received: 27 September 2018; Accepted: 8 November 2018; Published: 14 November 2018

Abstract: Neonatal screening programmes have been introduced in almost all European countries. In practice there are large differences, especially in the panel of conditions that are screened for, often without clear reasons. Policy making on a European level is lacking in contrast to the situation in the USA. Professionals have the knowledge to expand the panels but are dependent on policy-makers for the necessary funds. This paper is a call on the EU Commission to take up a role in providing equal access to neonatal screening for all children within the EU.

Keywords: (recommended) screening panel; policy making; harmonisation; patient advocacy

1. Introduction

Neonatal screening, in some countries called newborn screening (NBS), has been recognised as a valuable public health tool in many countries around the world. Based on the work by, e.g., Følling, Penrose and Centerwall in the 20th-century interbellum, Guthrie developed the first relatively easy and cheap assay for the identification of newborn children suffering from phenylketonuria [1]. In the following decade, the development of (radio)immunoassay systems opened the gate for the detection of blood components indicative of congenital hypothyroidism (CH) [2]. These two conditions were just the first of many more. Especially the development of the tandem mass spectrometry in the 1990s led to the possibility of high throughput screening of many newborn children for up to 40–50 different conditions [3,4].

It is self-evident that the implementation of an NBS programme based on modern technologies comes with a certain cost; the apparatus and the necessary manpower are relatively expensive, although this must also be seen in relation to the annual workload of each laboratory. In addition, so-called "multiplexing" methods as tandem mass spectrometry, facilitate the detection of more conditions without a substantial increase in running costs. On the other hand, most of the conditions in the screening panel, if undetected, very often lead to serious health problems, such as mental disabilities with concomitant high health care costs.

NBS is a clear example of a prevention programme with "cost before benefit". This notion should appeal to politicians and policy-makers in any country or jurisdiction. Everywhere money is tight and choices have to be made. An often-used framework for decision making are the criteria by Wilson and Jungner [5], which, even though they were published 50 years ago, are still valid today.

It would be ideal if policy-makers from different countries who are using these same criteria when judging how to structure their NBS programmes, could come to more or less the same conclusions whether or not to include a certain condition in their screening panel. In practice, this is not the case. Policy-makers give different "weights" to the various factors involved, such as who is the primary beneficiary of the screening system (baby/parent/society), how is the scientific evidence evaluated, and how is the system financed [6,7]. As a consequence, within Europe, the number of conditions screened for ranges from 1 (in Montenegro) to 35 (in Italy) [8–10].

Of course, it is understandable that poorer countries have less room for manoeuvring than richer countries. Moreover, the prevalence of a condition may vary, making it a good candidate in one country and an unlikely candidate in another; a well-known and often cited example is phenylketonuria (PKU), which hardly occurs in the Finnish population. Furthermore, the prevalence of certain conditions may increase over time, such as haemoglobinopathies, which have been part of the panels in Mediterranean countries since the 1990s. However, because of recent migration this prevalence is now so high that it was deemed appropriate to be included in the screening panels in the Netherlands, the U. and parts of Belgium.

Unfortunately, there is little interaction and discussion among policy-makers in various countries. Everyone is fixed on their own national situation. There is little willingness to accept the scientific data from other countries that indicate the net benefit of the inclusion of a condition in the screening panel. On the contrary, often the policy-makers require repetition of data collection by the medical professionals within their own country to satisfy the politicians before they decide.

Viewed from a distance, one could imagine that this situation would not apply to the member states of the European Union. After all, the EU, or at least its predecessors European Steel and Coal Community (ECSC) and European Economic (EEC), was established to facilitate interaction and collaboration between and among member states in many fields. The European Treaties have outlined how such collaboration should take place. Yet, health care has been a contentious topic. In the Maastricht and Amsterdam Treaties, Article 129.1 clearly states that *Community action, which shall complement national policies, shall be directed towards improving public health, preventing human illness and diseases, and obviating sources of danger to human health*. However, in the following paragraph, this has been limited immediately to an encouraging role only while leaving the initiative to the member states themselves (principle of subsidiarity): *The Community shall encourage cooperation between the Member States in the areas referred to in this Article and, if necessary, lend support to their action. Member States shall, in liaison with the Commission, coordinate among themselves their policies and programmes in the areas referred to in paragraph 1. The Commission may, in close contact with the Member States, take any useful initiative to promote such coordination. (Art 129.2)* [11,12]. This balancing act has been a major theme also in later EU documents on health care. See, for example, the European Committee of Experts in Rare Diseases (EUCERD) Opinion 2013 [13].

Therefore, for the neonatal screening community, the EU Council recommendations concerning rare diseases in 2009 came as a surprise [14]. Although it is focussed on rare diseases in general, it is very applicable to NBS since virtually all conditions in the NBS panels fall in the category of rare diseases. Subsequently, a call for tender was issued [15] that has led to the financing of an Executive Agency for Health and Concumers (EAHC)-project concerning the practices of newborn screening in European countries, within and outside the EU. The results have been published in a series of publications [16–18]. The Expert Opinion Document [18] has been submitted to the EU Commission that referred it to EUCERD. The conclusions of this committee have been documented [13]: Any subsequent action has been left to the member states.

Surprisingly, in other aspects of the fight against rare diseases, European wide collaboration appeared to be possible, such as the development of European Reference Networks (ERNs) in recent years. ERN's are centres of expertise with knowledge of only one or a limited number of rare diseases focussed on the treatment of patients. The intention is that within the EU, patients can be referred to an ERN even cross-border.

The question is why such collaboration among member states is possible at the back end of the process, i.e., treatment of identified individuals and not at the front end, i.e., the neonatal screening phase.

2. Achievements in the USA

As mentioned above neonatal screening started in the USA in the 1960s. To better judge the developing situation in Europe, and in particular in the European Union, it is informative to look at how NBS further developed and evolved in the USA. The USA has a federal government that in many aspects, including health, can give recommendations to the individual states that, in turn, can adopt them or not. Concerning NBS, until the 21st century, the States followed their own policy, based on their own appreciation of scientific evidence as well as learning from practical experience from other states. This led to large variations in the NBS systems between and among states. Some panels contained three conditions, others, more than 40 [19]. In 2002 the American College of Medical Genetics was commissioned to come up with *"recommendations focussed on newborn screening, including but not limited to the development of a uniform condition panel"*. The study, completed in 2005, led to a panel of 29 primary conditions, i.e., those that every state should screen for, and 25 secondary conditions, i.e., those that do not meet screening criteria but are identified anyway because the same markers are abnormal as in the primary conditions. The 29 were called the "recommended uniform screening panel" or RUSP.

The federal Secretary of Health adopted these recommendations. In the following years, the states harmonised their programmes such that every state now works towards full implementation of the RUSP.

New technical possibilities enabled further conditions to be picked up. To judge the value of such new developments a Secretary's Advisory Committee was created, issuing reports, based on which the RUSP was increased step by step, now comprising 35 conditions [20]. A protocol was developed to ascertain the scientific basis when considering further expansions of the RUSP [20].

3. Differences between the USA and Europe

Americans regard themselves as being an inhabitant of the country called the United States of America and can move around in the whole country. A recent estimate is that annually 10–25% of the population moves its household to another state [21]. Moreover, Americans have only a few common languages, English being the most prominent.

Europeans regard themselves as inhabitants of their own country and consider "Europe" to be far away, in the present time even more so than say 20 years ago. Moving around is much more restricted, although in principle there is free movement within the EU. Nevertheless, it is estimated that only 0.4% of European citizens move to another EU country [22]. In Europe, there is a multitude of languages, at least 40 or so.

These factors make Americans aware of what is going on elsewhere in their country, whereas Europeans, in general, have little or no idea of what is happening in neighbouring countries.

It has been mentioned above that in the USA the States receive recommendations from the federal government. In principle, they could ignore theses, but certainly, as regards to neonatal screening, this does not happen often. Parents- and advocacy-groups, such as March of Dimes and Save Babies through Screening, are very active and with a strong voice. They feel that it is unjustified if a newborn infant in State A is screened for a large number of conditions and in another state B for just a handful of conditions. They exert pressure via social networks and newspapers.

In Europe, there are also such advocacy groups, but they often work only within one country. On a European scale, there are umbrella organisations for professionals but not so many for advocacy groups. Thus, this diminishes the possibility of successful lobbying on a larger scale with politicians and policy-makers for harmonisation of neonatal screening panels.

4. The Way Forward in Europe and Especially within the EU

It is probably wishful thinking that the policy making concerning neonatal screening systems and the panel of screened conditions within Europe could be structured in a similar way as in the USA, at least within the next couple of years. EU Member States can always invoke the principle of subsidiarity if they are not inclined to collaborate. That should not prevent the EU Commission from strongly issuing recommendations, even if these are not adopted by all member states [23].

It could be argued that the European screening professionals should develop a "European RUSP" before calling upon action from the EU Commission. However, there seems to be no point in repeating what has been done elsewhere. NBS professionals already exchange views on who is doing what and share positive and negative experiences. The International Society for Neonatal Screening (ISNS), with members in almost all European countries as well as in many countries on other continents, facilitates these exchanges by frequently (co-)organising conferences, sending out monthly newsletters and providing information on its website. ISNS was very much involved in the above mentioned EAHC project [15]. ISNS recently teamed up with the International Patient Organisation for Primary Immunodeficiencies (IPOPI) to approach Commission officials as well as Members of the European Parliament to ask for attention for this topic.

It would be of value if patient and advocacy groups in the various countries would also join forces to convince policy-makers and politicians that collaboration saves time and money and that prevention through NBS is cheaper than treating unscreened patients who have developed clinical symptoms.

Finally, all European countries have ratified the UN Convention of the Rights of the Child [24]. Article 24 concerns the right to have optimal health care. Neonatal screening cannot solve all possible health problems, but it can certainly indicate which children in whatever country will need extra attention of the healthcare professionals.

It is high time that the European Commission instruct the Steering Group on health promotion, disease prevention and management of non-communicable diseases [25] to start work on this topic forthwith. The NBS professionals are ready to help!

Funding: This research received no external funding.

Acknowledgments: The author want to thanks Rodney R. Howell, Miami, USA, for helpful comments in the preparation of this manuscript.

Conflicts of Interest: The author declares no conflict of interest.

References

1. Guthrie, R.; Susi, A. A simple phenylalanine method for detecting phenylketonuria in large populations of newborn infants. *Pediatrics* **1963**, *32*, 338–343. [PubMed]
2. Dussault, J.H.; Laberge, C. Thyroxine (T4) determination by radioimmunological method in dried blood eluate: New diagnostic method of neonatal hypothyroidism? *Union Med. Can.* **1973**, *102*, 2062–2064. [PubMed]
3. Chace, D.H.; Millington, D.S.; Terada, N.; Kahler, S.G.; Roe, C.R.; Hofman, L.H. Rapid diagnosis of phenylketonuria by quantitative analysis of phenylalanine and tyrosine in neonatal blood spots using tandem mass spectrometry. *Clin. Chem.* **1993**, *39*, 66–71. [PubMed]
4. Rashed, M.S.; Rahbeeni, Z.; Ozand, P.T. Application of electrospray tandem mass spectrometry to neonatal screening. *Seminars Perinatol.* **1999**, *23*, 183–193. [CrossRef]
5. Wilson, J.M.; Jungner, Y.G. Principles and practice of mass screening for disease. *Bull. WHO* **1968**, *65*, 281–393.
6. Jansen, M.E.; Metternick-Jones, S.C.; Lister, K.J. International differences in the evaluation of conditions for newborn blood sot screening; a review of scientific literature and policy documents. *Eur. J. Hum. Genet.* **2016**, *25*, 10–16. [CrossRef] [PubMed]
7. Jansen, M.E.; Lister, K.J.; van Kranen, H.J.; Cornel, M.C. Policy making in newborn screening needs a structured and transparent approach. *Front. Public Health* **2017**, *5*, 53. [CrossRef] [PubMed]
8. Loeber, J.G. Neonatal screening in Europe; situation in 2004. *J. Inher. Metab. Dis.* **2007**, *30*, 430–438. [CrossRef] [PubMed]
9. Therrell, B.L.; Padilla, C.D.; Loeber, J.G.; Khneisser, I.; Saadallah, A.; Borrajo, G.J.C.; Adams, J. Current status of newborn screening worldwide 2015. *Seminars Perinatol.* **2015**, *39*, 171–187. [CrossRef] [PubMed]
10. Loeber, J.G. Status of neonatal screening in Europe revisited. in preparation.

11. Treaty on European Union, Signed at Maastricht on 7 February 1992. Off J Europ Commun 35: C191. Available online: http://eur-lex.europa.eu/legal-content/EN/TXT/PDF/?uri=OJ:C:1992:191:FULL&from=EN (accessed on 17 September 2018).
12. European Union. Treaty of Amsterdam, Off J Europ Commun 1997, ISBN 82-828-1652-46986. Available online: http://www.europarl.europa.eu/topics/treaty/pdf/amst-en.pdf (accessed on 17 September 2018).
13. EUCERD Opinion 2013 Newborn Screening in Europe; Opinion of the EUCERD on Potential Areas for European Collaboration. Available online: http://www.eucerd.eu/wp-content/uploads/2013/07/EUCERD_NBS_Opinion_Adopted.pdf (accessed on 17 September 2018).
14. EU Council Recommendation of 8 June 2009 on an action in the field of rare diseases (2009/C 151/02). Available online: http://ec.europa.eu/chafea/documents/health/prague-rd-council-recommendation_en.pdf (accessed on 17 September 2018).
15. EU-Executive Agency for Health and Consumers. Call for Tender "Evaluation of Population Newborn Screening Practices for Rare Disorders in Member States of the European Union" EHC/2009/Health/09. Available online: http://old.iss.it/binary/cnmr4/cont/TechnicalSpecifications.pdf (accessed on 17 September 2018).
16. Loeber, J.G.; Burgard, P.; Cornel, M.C.; Rigter, T.; Weinreich, S.S.; Rupp, K.; Hoffmann, G.F.; Vittozzi, L. Newborn screening programmes in Europe; arguments and efforts regarding harmonization. Part 1–From blood spot to screening result. *J. Inher. Metab. Dis.* **2012**, *35*, 603–611. [CrossRef] [PubMed]
17. Burgard, P.; Rupp, K.; Lindner, M.; Haege, G.; Rigter, T.; Weinreich, S.S.; Loeber, J.G.; Taruscio, D.; Vittozzi, L.; Cornel, M.C.; et al. Newborn screening programmes in Europe; arguments and efforts regarding harmonization. Part 2–From screening laboratory results to treatment, follow-up and quality assurance. *J. Inher. Metab. Dis.* **2012**, *35*, 613–625. [CrossRef] [PubMed]
18. Cornel, M.C.; Rigter, T.; Weinreich, S.S.; Burgard, P.; Hoffmann, G.F.; Lindner, M.; Loeber, J.G.; Rupp, K.; Taruscio, D.; Vittozzi, L. Expert Opinion document Newborn screening in Europe. Based on the EU Tender "Evaluation of population newborn screening practices for rare disorders in Member States of the European Union". *Eur. J. Hum. Genet.* **2014**, *22*, 12–17.
19. Watson, M.S.; Mann, M.Y.; Lloyd-Puryear, M.A.; Rinaldo, P.; Howell, R.R. Newborn screening: Toward a uniform screening panel and system—Executive summary. *Pediatrics* **2006**, *117*, S296–S307. [CrossRef] [PubMed]
20. Advisory Committee on Heritable Disorders in Newborns and Children. Available online: https://www.hrsa.gov/advisory-committees/heritable-disorders/rusp/index.html (accessed on 13 September 2018).
21. Avric. Available online: http://avrickdirect.com/homedata/?p=31 (accessed on 17 September 2018).
22. Eurostat. Available online: https://ec.europa.eu/eurostat/statistics-explained/index.php/Migration_and_migrant_population_statistics/nl (accessed on 17 September 2018).
23. Anonymous. Addressing the high burden and significant unmet needs in phenylketonuria (PKU). In Proceedings of the European Parliament Policy Roundtable, Brussels, Belgium, 11 July 2018; p. 6.
24. UN Convention of the Rights of the Child. Available online: https://www.ohchr.org/en/professionalinterest/pages/crc.aspx (accessed on 17 September 2018).
25. EU Steering Group on Health Promotion. Disease Prevention and Management of Non-Communicable Diseases. Available online: https://ec.europa.eu/health/non_communicable_diseases/steeringgroup_promotionprevention_en (accessed on 18 September 2018).

 © 2018 by the author. Licensee MDPI, Basel, Switzerland. This article is an open access article distributed under the terms and conditions of the Creative Commons Attribution (CC BY) license (http://creativecommons.org/licenses/by/4.0/).

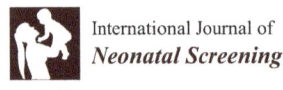

Review

Sickle Cell Disease—Genetics, Pathophysiology, Clinical Presentation and Treatment

Baba P. D. Inusa [1,*], Lewis L. Hsu [2], Neeraj Kohli [3], Anissa Patel [4], Kilali Ominu-Evbota [5], Kofi A. Anie [6] and Wale Atoyebi [7]

1. Paediatric Haematology, Evelina London Children's Hospital, Guy's and St Thomas NHS Trust, London SE1 7EH, UK
2. Pediatric Hematology-Oncology, University of Illinois at Chicago, Chicago, IL 60612, USA; LewHsu@uic.edu
3. Haematology, Guy's and St Thomas NHS Trust, London SE1 7EH, UK; Neeraj.Kohli@gstt.nhs.uk
4. Holborn Medical Centre, GP, London WC1N 3NA, UK; Anissa.patel@nhs.net
5. Paediatrics Department, Basildon and Thurrock University Hospitals, NHS Foundation Trust, Basildon SS16 5NL, UK; Kilali.ominu-evbota@btuh.nhs.uk
6. Haematology and Sickle Cell Centre, London North West University Healthcare NHS Trust, London NW10 7NS, UK; kofi.anie@nhs.net
7. Department of Clinical Haematology, Cancer and Haematology Centre, Oxford University Hospitals NHS Foundation Trust, Churchill Hospital, Oxford OX3 9DU, UK; Wale.atoyebi@ouh.nhs.uk
* Correspondence: Baba.inusa@gstt.nhs.uk

Received: 16 February 2019; Accepted: 24 April 2019; Published: 7 May 2019

Abstract: Sickle cell disease (SCD) is a monogenetic disorder due to a single base-pair point mutation in the β-globin gene resulting in the substitution of the amino acid valine for glutamic acid in the β-globin chain. Phenotypic variation in the clinical presentation and disease outcome is a characteristic feature of the disorder. Understanding the pathogenesis and pathophysiology of the disorder is central to the choice of therapeutic development and intervention. In this special edition for newborn screening for haemoglobin disorders, it is pertinent to describe the genetic, pathologic and clinical presentation of sickle cell disease as a prelude to the justification for screening. Through a systematic review of the literature using search terms relating to SCD up till 2019, we identified relevant descriptive publications for inclusion. The scope of this review is mainly an overview of the clinical features of pain, the cardinal symptom in SCD, which present following the drop in foetal haemoglobin as young as five to six months after birth. The relative impact of haemolysis and small-vessel occlusive pathology remains controversial, a combination of features probably contribute to the different pathologies. We also provide an overview of emerging therapies in SCD.

Keywords: sickle cell disease (SCD); pathophysiology; hydroxyurea/hydroxycarbamide; haemolysis; vaso-occlusive crisis; acute chest syndrome; end-organ damage; bone marrow transplant; anaemia; foetal haemoglobin; gene therapy for haemoglobinopathies

---

1. Introduction

Sickle cell disease (SCD) was first reported by Herrick in 1910 even though reports suggest prior description of the disorder [1]; it is the result of homozygous and compound heterozygote inheritance of a mutation in the *β-globin* gene. A single base-pair point mutation (GAG to GTG) results in the substitution of the amino acid glutamic acid (hydrophilic) to Valine (hydrophobic) in the 6th position of the β-chain of haemoglobin referred to as haemoglobin S (HbS) [2]. Phenotypic variation in clinical presentation is a unique feature of SCD despite a well-defined Mendelian inheritance, the first to be molecularly characterised as described by Pauling [3] and confirmed to be due to a single amino acid substitution by Ingram [3] almost 70 years ago. SCD is a multi-organ, multi-system disorder with both acute and chronic complications presenting when foetal haemoglobin (HbF) drops towards the adult level by five to six months of age [4].

2. Classification

The inheritance of homozygous HbS otherwise referred to as sickle cell anaemia (SCA) is the most predominant form of SCD, the proportion varies according the country of origin [5–7]. The next most common form of SCD is the co-inheritance of HbS and HbC—referred to as HbSC, this is most prevalent in Western Africa, particularly Burkina Fasso and Mali and the coastal countries including Ghana, Benin and Western Nigeria [5,7,8]. The co-inheritance with β thalassaemia results in a sickle β thalassaemia genotype (*HbS/βo or HbS/β+*), depending on the genetic lesion on the thalassaemia component, the clinical presentation may be mild or equally as severe as homozygous SCD (HbS/HbS) [9]. Those with *HbS/βo*-thalassaemia have a more severe course of disease similar to homozygous SS patients, while offspring with *HbS/β+*-thalassaemia depending on the β-globin mutation is associated with variable phenotype from mild to severe phenotypes SCD [3,10].

3. Epidemiology

SCD is one of the most common inherited life-threatening disorders in human, it predominantly affect people of African, Indiana and Arab ancestry [5,11,12]. It is estimated that over 80% of over 300,000 annual births occur in sub-Saharan Africa (SSA), the largest burden from Nigeria and Democratic Republic of Congo [13]. The gene frequency is highest in West African countries with 1 in 4 to 3 (25–30%) being carriers of HbS compared to 1/400 African Americans and is variable in European populations [14–16]. The prevalence of SCD in developed countries is increasing partly due to migration from high prevalent countries [17–20]. It is estimated that over 14,000 people live with SCD in the UK, similar to France, while countries like Italy, Germany have seen increasing numbers from Africa [21–24]. With increasing survival, the age distribution of SCD is changing from a childhood disorder pattern that patients now survive into adulthood and old age. It is now reported that over 94% of those born with SCD now survive into adulthood in the US, France and UK in contrast to the high mortality in SSA where 50–90% may die in the first five years of life [12,25,26]. In low resource settings and countries where newborn screening is not yet standard care, patients may die young even before diagnosis is confirmed [27]. Among the common causes of death in the absence of early diagnosis followed by education and preventive therapies such as penicillin prophylaxis and regular surveillance include infections, severe anaemia (acute splenic sequestration, aplastic anaemia) and multi-organ failure [28]. It is essential therefore that Newborn and Early Infant diagnosis is given the priority it deserves by those countries where SCD is a public health problem [28,29]. The implementation of early infant diagnosis remains out of reach for the majority of countries in SSA despite multiple declarations by international organisations and public statements by politicians to honour such commitments. The benefits for screening can only become meaningful when such practice is embraced by policy-makers across the continent and India where the majority of SCD are born and live. Comprehensive care includes penicillin V prophylaxis, Hydroxycarbamide therapy and preventive therapies such as antimalarials and health promotion where relevant will improve outcomes and health related quality of life [30].

4. Pathophysiology

The schematic representation in Figure 1 highlights the pathophysiology of SCD [31]. Red blood cells (RBCs) that contain HbS or HbS in combination with other abnormal β alleles, when exposed to deoxygenated environment undergo polymerisation and become rigid. The rigid RBC's are liable to haemolysis, and due to increased density may affect blood flow and endothelial vessel wall integrity. The dense rigid RBC's lead to vaso-occlusion, tissue ischaemia, infarction as well as haemolysis [32]. The consequence of haemolysis is a complex cascade of events including nitric oxide consumption; haemolysis linked nitric oxide dysregulation and endothelial dysfunction which underlie complications such as leg ulceration, stroke, pulmonary hypertension and priapism [33]. Unlike normal RBC's with half-life of approximately 120 days, sickle RBC's (sRBC) may survive just 10–20 days due to increased haemolysis [34]. During deoxygenation; healthy haemoglobin rearranges itself into a different conformation, enabling binding with carbon dioxide molecules which reverts to normal when released [32]. In contrast, HbS tends to polymerise into rigid insoluble strands and tactoids, which are gel-like substances containing Hb crystals. During acute sickling, intravascular haemolysis results in free haemoglobin in the serum, while RBC's gaining Na^+, Ca^{2+} with corresponding loss of K^+ [31]. The increase in the concentration of Ca^{2+} leads to dysfunction in the calcium pump. The calcium depends on ATPase but it is unclear what role calcium plays in membrane rigidity attributed to cytoskeletal membrane interactions. [35]. Furthermore, hypoxia also inhibits the production of nitric oxide, thereby causing the adhesion of sickle cells to the vascular endothelium [33]. The lysis of erythrocytes leads to increase in extracellular haemoglobin, thus increasing affinity and binding to available nitric oxide or precursors of nitric oxide; thereby reducing its levels and further contributing to vasoconstriction [32].

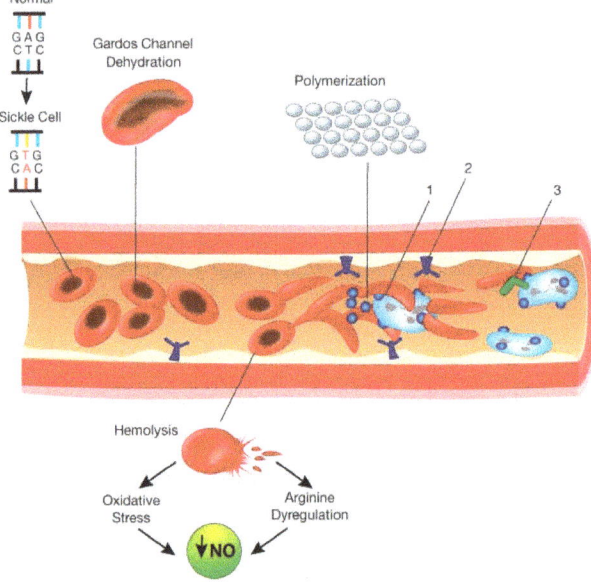

Figure 1. Schematic representation of the pathophysiology (in part) of sickle cell anemia. A single gene mutation (GAG→GTG and CTC→CAC) results in a defective haemoglobin that when exposed to de-oxygenation (depicted in the right half of the diagram) polymerizes (upper right of the diagram), resulting in the formation of sickle cells. Vaso-occlusion can then occur. The disorder is also characterized by abnormal adhesive properties of sickle cells; peripheral blood mononuclear cells (depicted in light blue; shown as the large cells under the sickle cells) and platelets (depicted in dark blue; shown as the dark circular shapes on the mononuclear cells) adhere to the sickled erythrocytes. This aggregate is labelled 1. The mononuclear cells have receptors (e.g., CD44 (labeled 3 and depicted in dark green on the cell surface)) that bind to ligands, such as P-selectin (labeled 2 and shown on the endothelial surface), that are unregulated. The sickle erythrocytes can also adhere directly to the endothelium. Abnormal movement or rolling and slowing of cells in the blood also can occur. These changes result in endothelial damage. The sickled red cells also become dehydrated as a result of abnormalities in the Gardos channel. Hemolysis contributes to oxidative stress and dysregulation of arginine metabolism, both of which lead to a decrease in nitric oxide (NO) that, in turn, contributes to the vasculopathy that characterizes SCD.

5. Disease Modifiers

The sickle β-globin mutation renders the sickle gene pleiotropic in nature, with variable phenotypic expression associated with complex genetic and environmental interactions, as well as disease modifiers that are increasingly being recognised. Sickle RBC (sRBC) polymerisation in deoxygenated environments is influenced by a number of factors including the co-inheritance of alpha thalassaemia, foetal haemoglobin (HbF) level which is determined by a number of genetic factors including genetic variations of BLC11A, HBS1L-MYB and HBB loci and hydroxycarbamide therapy amongst others [35]. The BCL11A and ZBTB7A genes (LRF protein) are responsible for the suppression of γ chains, and HbF production. HbF reduces sickle cell polymerisation due to reduction in HbS concentration and the fact that it is excluded from the sickle cell polymers. HbF also has high oxygen retention thereby ameliorating both the vaso-occlusive and haemolytic pathology in SCD. Among the four main sickle haplotypes, the level of HbF is highest in the Indian/Arab haplotype [8] predominantly found in the Arab Peninsula and India followed by the Senegal, and Benin haplotypes most predominant in Sub-Saharan Africa. The Bantu haplotype with the lowest HbF is predominantly found in Central African countries [8,36]. Alpha thalassaemia also modulates the expression of SCD. People with one or two α genes deleted have less haemolysis and fewer vasculopathy complications [8].

6. Clinical Manifestations

SCD is characterised by protean manifestations ranging from acute generalised pain to early onset stroke, leg ulcers and the risk of premature deaths from multi-organ failure [8]. As a result of the effect of HbF, clinical features do not begin until the middle to second part of the first year of post-natal life when this has predominantly switched to adult haemoglobin [36–40].

6.1. Vaso-Occlusive Crisis (Pain)

Patients with SCD may experience intense pain early in infancy, childhood and adulthood. Pain usually accounts for the majority of hospitalisations and overall negative impact in patients' health related quality of life. Pain is the cardinal feature of SCD and it is characteristically unpredictable, episodic in nature, described as one of the most excruciating forms of pain that affects human beings. Pain occurs due to stimulation of nociceptive nerve fibres caused by microvascular occlusion. The microcirculation is obstructed by sRBCs, thereby restricting the flow of blood to the organ and this results in (i) ischaemia, (ii) oedema, (iii) pain, (iv) necrosis, and (v) organ damage [10]. In the first year of life one of the cardinal features is the 'hand-foot syndrome' due to vaso-occlusion of post-capillary vasculature resulting in tissue oedema and pain of the extremities [41]. Infants display their pain nonverbally with irritability and apparent 'regression' tendencies such as inability to weight bear, walk or crawl. In older children and adults, vaso-occlusive pain can affect any part of the body. The onset of pain is spontaneous, usually no precipitating factors; well-known triggers include infections, fever, dehydration, acidosis, sudden change in weather including wind speed, cold, rain and air pollution. Resolution of pain is unpredictable. Acute pain might lead to chronic pain [42].

6.2. Anaemia

Symptomatic anaemia is the commonest symptom in SCD generally more common in SCA (Homozygous S), which usually runs the lowest haemoglobin level common to double heterozygous states. The steady state haemoglobin for asymptomatic patients varies according to the phenotype, ranging from levels as low as 60–80 g/L for homozygous S and /Sβo to 100–110 g/L in double heterozygous SC and Sβ+ forms. However, the rate of fall from individual steady state haemoglobin level may trigger symptoms of hypoxia (aplastic crises) or a shock-like state (e.g., acute splenic sequestration) [4,43].

6.3. Acute Aplastic Crisis

The most common cause of acquired bone marrow failure in SCD and other haemolytic disorders is caused by Parvovirus B19 [44]. This virus causes the fifth disease and normally in healthy children is quite mild, associated with malaise, fever and sometimes a mild rash; the virus affects erythropoiesis by invading progenitors of RBCs in the bone marrow and destroying them, thus preventing new RBCs from being made. There's a slight drop in haematocrit in children with HbAA who are generally unaffected, however in SCD as the lifespan of RBC's is reduced to about 10–20 days, there is a significant drop in haemoglobin concentration. Parvovirus B19 infection usually takes about four days to one week to resolve and patients with SCD usually require a blood transfusion [39,44].

6.4. Infection

SCD increases susceptibility to infections, notably bacterial sepsis and malaria in children under five years [45]. Respiratory infections can trigger the sickle-cell acute chest syndrome, with a high risk of death. Risk factors for infections include: (i) functional asplenia/hyposplenia which present with reduced splenic immune response at a very young age, (ii) impaired fixation of complement, (iii) reduced oxidative burst capacity of chronically activated neutrophils, dysfunctional IgM and IgG antibody responses and defective opsonisation. The main pathogen of concern is *Streptococcus pneumoniae*, though severe and systemic infections arise with *Haemophilus influenzae*, *Neisseria meningitides*, and *Salmonellae* leads to osteomyelitis especially *Salmonella* due to bowel ischaemia and gut flora dissemination [46,47].

6.5. Splenic Sequestration Crisis

The main function of the spleen is the removal of defective red blood cells including sickled RBCs (sRBC) resulting in further haemolysis [48]. Blood flow through the spleen is slow reducing oxygen tension and increased polymerisation in HbS. As a result of the narrow capillaries in the splenic vascular bed, further hypoxia occurs with RBC polymerisation and entrapment of affected blood cells. This leads to a cycle of hypoxia, RBC polymerisation, and reduced blood flow causing the spleen to enlarge, for unexplained reasons, this may occur suddenly with pooling of blood within the vascular bed resulting in shock and circulatory failure. The rapidly increasing spleen size may lead to abdominal distension, sudden weakness, increased thirst, tachycardia and tachypnoea. Splenic sequestration crisis is an emergency because if left untreated, it can lead to death in 1–2 h due to circulatory failure [49].

6.6. Other Complications

The complications listed above are highlighted as those affecting babies and young children, because these are immediately relevant after newborn screening. Older children, adolescents, and young adults develop many chronic complications: stroke, cognitive dysfunction, priapism, leg ulcers, avascular necrosis (of the femoral head or humeral head), chronic pain, retinopathy, pulmonary hypertension, acute kidney injury, chronic kidney disease, thromboembolic events, and hepatic sequestration [50,51], cholelithiasis (gallstones) and cholecystitis as a result of excessive production and precipitation of bilirubin due to haemolysis. SCD also increases susceptibility to complications in pregnancy [52].

6.7. Psychosocial Impact

SCD has a significant psychosocial impact on patients and families [53]. This mainly results from the effect of pain and symptoms on their daily lives, and society's attitudes towards them. Cultural factors are particularly important to these problems because of beliefs and practices [54]. Furthermore, the ability of people with SCD to cope with their condition varies greatly because severity, general health, and quality of life varies greatly among individuals [55,56].

7. Treatment and Management

SCD causes a range of acute and long-term complications, requiring a multi-disciplinary approach, involving various medical specialists. In the United Kingdom, comprehensive SCD care is coordinated by specialist haemoglobinopathy teams [57]. Such teams play a key role in education about SCD for patients and their families, as well as guiding treatment with disease-modifying therapies, access to psychology, social and welfare support. Additionally, they coordinate screening services such as Transcranial Doppler (TCD) ultrasound monitoring in children, detection of iron overload or allo-antibody formation in individuals on transfusion programmes, and referral to specialists for major organ complications with an interest in SCD.

8. Management of Acute Vaso-Occlusive Crises (Pain)

Pain is the commonest acute complication of SCD, and significantly impact health-related quality of life [58]. Pain management may vary from patient to patient depending on family dynamics and individual patient thresholds or access to health care, however mild to moderate painful episodes may be treated in the home without the need of attending a health facility. Self-help psychological strategies including distraction techniques such as guided imagery can be a useful evidence-based adjunct to managing pain, and patients who utilise complementary coping strategies tend to require fewer hospitalisations [53,59]. The management strategy for pain includes 4 stages: which are assessment, treatment, reassessment, and adjustment [60]. It is also important to take into consideration (1) the severity of pain and (2) the patient's past response to different analgesics and to follow their regular protocols to alleviate the patient's pain.

Supportive Care

Given the fact that pain is often triggered by infection, exposure to cold or dehydration, supportive care during these episodes involves providing hydration, warmth and treating any treating the underlying infection. Simple devices such as incentive spirometry can be critical in preventing complications such as acute chest syndrome. Longer-term infection prevention varies regionally but can involve vaccination programs and penicillin prophylaxis [61].

9. Disease Modifying and Curative Treatments

Currently the only available disease-modifying medications for SCD are hydroxycarbamide and L-glutamine. Both are given daily to reduce the rate of acute complications, but results vary from person to person. Another effective disease modifying therapy is blood transfusion to raise the haemoglobin for improved oxygenation in severe anaemia and also to reduce the proportion of sickle haemoglobin (HbS%) may be give as a simple top-up blood transfusion or as exchange transfusion (manual or automated). The main curative therapy is stem cell transplantation while gene therapy is in the horizon in clinical Trials.

9.1. Hydroxycarbamide

Hydroxycarbamide has gained widely accepted use globally [62]. Although it was originally used as a cytoreductive agent by inhibiting ribonucleotide reductase, the main mechanism through which hydroxycarbamide works in SCD is through increasing total haemoglobin concentration and HbF production [63]. Hydroxycarbamide also reduces the number of leucocytes in blood, and reduces expression of surface adhesion molecules on neutrophils, red cells and vascular endothelium resulting in improved blood flow and reducing vaso-occlusion [62]. A number of trials in adults and children have shown beneficial effects of long-term hydroxycarbamide use, including reducing the severity and frequency of crisis in children with SCD [64]. The Multi-Centre Study of Hydroxycarbamide (MSH) showed that over a two-year follow-up period, adults on hydroxycarbamide had a significantly lower frequency of painful crises compared with placebo (median 2.5 versus 4.5 respectively, $p = 0.001$), as well as lower incidence of acute chest syndrome (25 versus 51, $p = 0.001$) and lower need for blood transfusion (48 patients versus 73, $p = 0.001$). A subsequent observational study following up on participants of the MSH study over a nine-year period showed a 40% reduction in mortality amongst patients on hydroxycarbamide. Patients with SCD who have increased HbF levels suffer less pain and live longer [62]. A meta-analysis in 2007 looked at effectiveness, efficacy and toxicity of hydroxycarbamide in children with SCD and they found that HbF levels increased by about 10% and also found a significant increase in haemoglobin concentration by approximately 1%; and on average there was a decrease in hospitalisation rates by 71% as well as a decrease in the frequency of pain crisis [62,65]. Indications for Hydroxycarbamide vary according to the phenotype, age and individual practice [65]. The US National Institute of Health (NIH) evidence-based guidelines and British Society of Haematology recommend offering Hydroxycarbamide to all HbSS and HbS/β0 thalassaemia genotype children from age of 1 year even though actual practice varies widely between continents.

In adults, indications for hydroxycarbamide may include [66–68]:

1. Frequent painful episodes (>3 per annum) or chronic debilitating pain not controlled by usual protocols.
2. History of stroke or a high risk for stroke or other severe vaso-occlusive events.
3. Severe symptomatic anaemia.
4. History of acute chest syndrome.

Patients on hydroxycarbamide undergo regular monitoring for the development of leucopenia and/or thrombocytopenia. Hydroxycarbamide can cause birth defects in animal models, hence the caution about its use during pregnancy, but hydroxycarbamide has not yet been linked to birth defects in humans. Short term research has shown only minor side effects and the benefits of using hydroxycarbamide outweigh any short-term adverse effects [62,65].

9.2. L-Glutamine

Glutamine is a conditionally essential amino acid, meaning that although the body normally makes sufficient amounts, at times of stress the body's need for glutamine increases, and in such instances, it also relies on dietary glutamine to meet this demand. The U.S. Food and Drug Administration (FDA) approved use of pharmaceutical-grade L-glutamine for sickle patients aged five years or older in July 2017 [69]. Formal clinical trials showed that this purified version of glutamine significantly reduced the frequency of acute complications of SCD. Side effects appear to be minor and do not require lab monitoring [31,69].

FDA approval was based on the results of two double-blind randomized placebo-controlled trials studying the effect of L-glutamine on clinical end-points in adults and children over five years old with HbSS or *HbS/βo* thalassaemia. A phase III double-blind placebo-controlled trial randomising two hundred and thirty patients aged 5 to 58 years in a 2:1 ratio to either 0.3 g/kg oral L-glutamine twice daily, rounded to 5 g doses to a maximum of 30 g, or placebo. Concerns around the study results are due to the high dropout rate, with 97 (63.8%) participants in the intervention group and 59 (75.6%) in the placebo group completing the eleven-month study. The researchers showed a 17.9% reduction in the mean frequency of sickle crises in the L-glutamine group (3.2 versus 3.9 in the L-glutamine and placebo groups respectively ($p = 0.0152$)) and significantly fewer pain crises in the L-glutamine group (median 3.0 in the L-glutamine group and 4.0 in the placebo group, $p = 0.005$). There was significantly fewer hospitalisations in the L-glutamine group (median 2.0 in the L-glutamine group and 3.0 in the placebo group, $p = 0.005$) [69]. There were also significant reductions in the frequency of acute chest crises (8.6% on the L-glutamine group versus 23.1% in the placebo group, $p = 0.003$), and duration of hospital admissions (median 6.5 in the L-glutamine group versus 11 in the placebo group, $p = 0.02$) [69]. Potential concerns around use include the lack of long-term follow up data, financial cost compared with hydroxycarbamide, and theoretical concern around reducing treatment concordance with hydroxycarbamide therapy amongst patients seeking more naturalistic medication [70].

9.3. Blood Transfusion

Individuals with SCD have a baseline level of anaemia due to their chronic haemolysis. Blood transfusions are not given to correct this baseline anaemia or for acute pain episodes. Instead, transfusions are given to correct acute severe anaemia where the haemoglobin falls significantly below that individual's baseline, and the resulting impairment in oxygen delivery to body tissues would otherwise propagate further sickling of deoxygenated Hb. Examples include red cell aplasia caused by Parvovirus B19 infection, acute splenic sequestration or hyperhaemolysis crises [71]. In an acute setting, transfusion is also used to bridge periods of severe physiologic stress like major surgery or critical illness including acute chest crises. In this setting, blood transfusion with HbS-negative blood reduces the proportion of circulating haemoglobin that is able to sickle, and hence reducing vessel occlusion and haemolysis from abnormal sickle RBCs. Long-term transfusions are instituted as a disease-modifying treatment in specific situations, such as to prevent stroke. The issues that arise as a result of long term transfusion complications include: (i) Allo-immunization, where after receiving a blood transfusion an individual develops antibodies to an antigen on the transfused red cells, which can increase the risk of having haemolytic reactions to blood that they are transfused in future; (ii) Iron overload, although treatment of iron overload is becoming more tolerable with the new oral chelators and, (iii) Risk of transfusion-transmitted infections, especially in countries where only limited screening of donated blood is available [39,72].

9.4. Bone Marrow Transplantation (BMT)

BMT is the only current cure for SCD and is one of the newer methods of treatments available. Results indicate an event-free survival rate of approximately 91% and a mortality rate of less than 5% [51]. BMT carries significant risks, such as the new bone marrow producing leucocytes attacking hosts tissue cells which is known as Graft-versus-host-disease (GVHD) [73]. Tissues affected include skin, liver, gastrointestinal tract and eyes, symptoms include nausea, weight loss and jaundice. The risk of developing GVHD is low when the donor and the recipient are related and matched for HLA type. When the donor and recipient aren't related or there is a mismatch in HLA types, there is greater the likelihood of developing GVHD; strategies for careful immunosuppression after transplant can reduce the risk of GVHD [74]. Other risks from undergoing BMT include strokes, fatal infection, organ damage, and fits. Thus, BMT requires specialist centres with highly experienced teams and advanced technological resources. Due to the current levels of risk, a bone marrow transplant is only usually recommended if the symptoms and complications of SCD are severe enough to warrant the risks of BMT [75].

10. New and Emerging Therapies for Sickle Cell Disease

Researchers are studying several novel and existing medicines for SCD, in order to address different pathophysiological mechanisms. Candidates in the "pipeline" of clinical studies include adhesion blockers, HbS polymerization blockers, antioxidants, regulators of inflammation and activation, and promoters for nitric oxide. Developing a range of mechanistic targets may allow combination therapies to be developed, both to prevent and to treat acute sickle cell complications. For this reason, many phase II and III studies have included patients already established on hydroxycarbamide, to see if combination treatments can provide additional benefit. Examples of some of the key agents under investigation are discussed below.

10.1. Treatments that Reduce HbS Polymerisation

GBT440 (Voxelotor) is an oral small molecule designed to increase the oxygen affinity of HbS, shifting the oxygen dissociation curve of oxy-HbS to the left [76]. It does this by reversibly binding with the N-terminal valine of alpha (α) chain of Haemoglobin, changing its conformational structure and stabilizing the oxygenation form of the molecule. This reduces the concentration of deoxygenated

HbS, which is the form of the molecule that polymerises to give the sickle phenotype. An initial phase I/II study showed Voxelotor to be well tolerated, with predictable pharmacodynamics and pharmacokinetics [76].

10.2. Nutritional Supplements

Omega-3 fatty acids have been purified from fish oil and tested for benefits as antioxidant, antithrombotic, and anti-inflammatory benefit. The clinical trials have used products with different purity, different proportions of types of omega-3 fatty acids, and different dosages. A trial in Georgia showed significantly decreased pain and decreased platelet activation in adults with sickle cell anemia on large daily quantities of fish oil capsules compared to adults on large daily quantities of olive oil capsules as placebo control [31,77,78]. A large trial in Sudan showed school absences were significantly decreased in children with sickle cell anemia taking fish oil compared to those taking placebo [77].

Folic acid is widely prescribed for SCD with the rationale that increased erythropoiesis causes increased risk of folate deficiency. A Cochrane Review evaluated the one double-blinded placebo-controlled clinical trial that was conducted in the 1980's and concluded that the trial presents mixed evidence of benefit in children and no trials were found in adults [79]. Although the Cochrane reviewers recommend further investigation, they also state that no further trials of folic acid in SCD are expected [79].

EvenFlo, an herbal mixture marketed online by Healing Blends, is the only one of several herbal supplements to begin clinical trials. An open-label observational study was published online by the company in 2017 [78] and https://healingblendsglobal.com/2017/02/clinical-study-evenflo/. A randomized controlled trial was recently completed and submitted for peer reviewed publication, still pending at the time of this writing.

A traditional herbal product used to treat SCD in Nigeria, Niprisan, showed promising pre-clinical data although it is likely to have drug interactions from its significant inhibition of cytochrome CYP3A4 activity. Niprisan was awarded "Orphan Drug Status" by the FDA [32,80]. However, financial barriers halted production and Niprisan has not progressed to clinical trials [81].

10.3. Agents that Reduce Cell Adhesion to Activated Microvascular Endothelium: Targeted Selectin Inhibitors (Crizanlizumab, Rivipansel, Heparins and Heparin-Derived Molecules)

Selectins are transmembrane glycoproteins that are important for cell trafficking for the innate immune system, lymphocytes and platelets. Different families of selectins are expressed on endothelial cells, leucocytes and platelets. Leucocyte rolling and tethering by P and E-selectin, expressed on the surface of activated microvascular endothelium may contribute to reduced blood flow velocity and increased sickling and vaso-occlusion. Therefore, targeted P-selectin inhibitors (Crizanlizumab (SEG101, previously SELG1)), pan-selectin inhibitors (Rivipansel/GMI-1070) have undergone phase II trials. Crizanlizumab was evaluated in a double-blind, randomized, placebo-controlled phase II trial which assigned participants aged 16 to 65 years to either low-dose intravenous Crizanlizumab (2.5 mg/kg), high-dose intravenous Crizanlizumab (5.0 mg/kg), or placebo, administered over 30 min, 14 times throughout the course of one year. Results showed that a 43 percent relative risk reduction in annual acute pain episodes (1.63 vs. 2.98) occurred when comparing the high-dose Crizanlizumab and placebo treatment groups ($p = 0.01$). Not only did the therapy decrease the annual acute pain episode rate, but the high dose of Crizanlizumab also delayed the first and second acute pain episodes when compared with placebo (first episode, 4.07 months vs. 1.38 months, $p = 0.001$; second episode, 10.32 months vs. 5.09 months, $p = 0.02$; respectively [31,82].

Heparins are able to bind selectins and it has been posited that this allows heparins to reduce sickle cell adhesion to activated endothelium. A double-blind placebo-controlled randomised trial reported a statistically significant reduction in duration of painful crisis and duration of hospital admission with use of tinzaparin, a low molecular weight heparin, compared with supportive care only, amongst 253 patients with SCD admitted with acute painful crisis. Sevuparin is a novel heparin-derived compound in which the anticoagulant effect has been removed, but which retains the selectin-binding effect of heparins [83,84].

10.4. Agents that Improve Blood Flow through Anticoagulant Effect: Antiplatelet and Anticoagulant Agents

10.4.1. Prasugrel

Prasugrel inhibits ADP-mediated platelet aggregation. Previous research suggested that activated platelets adhere to endothelium during vaso-occlusive episodes and recruit leucocytes. A phase III study of 341 children with SCD did not show a significant reduction in vaso-occlusive events per person-year in children taking Prasugrel compared with those taking placebo. It also did not show a significant reduction in diary-reported pain events [85,86].

10.4.2. Apixaban

Apixaban is an oral direct Factor Xa inhibitor, which therefore prevents the activation of prothrombin to thrombin. A phase III randomised placebo-controlled trial is underway investigating the effectiveness of prophylactic dose Apixaban at reducing mean daily pain scores in adults with SCD [87].

10.5. Agents that Restore Depleted Nitric Oxide within the Microvasculature: Statins, L-Arginine, PDE9

Nitric oxide released from endothelium promotes vessel smooth muscle relaxation, resulting in vasodilatation and improved blood flow. It also suppresses platelet aggregation, as well as reducing expression of cell adhesion molecules on endothelium and reducing release of procoagulant factors. Intravascular haemolysis results in release of free haemoglobin into the patient's plasma [63]. This acts as a nitric oxide scavenger. In addition, arginase released from lysed red cells breaks down arginine, which is a substrate used to make endogenous nitric oxide. Both these events result in depletion of nitric oxide levels. Two drug groups that have been investigated for their effect on improving nitric oxide reserves in SCD are statins and L-arginine. Statins inhibit Rho kinase resulting in endothelial nitric oxide synthase activation [35,88].

10.6. Gene Therapy

Gene therapy is in early studies as a possible cure for sickle cell anaemia. The approach is based on stem cells and gene therapy; instead of using embryonic stem cells, host stem cells are derived by manipulating and reprogramming cells from patient's own blood cells with genetic engineering used to correct the inborn genetic error. Because the cells are provided by the patient, there is no need to find another person to serve as a donor of stem cells and there should be no risk of GVHD. The aim is to transform a patient's blood cells into pluripotent stem cells and replace the defective portion of the gene. These cells will then be coaxed into becoming hematopoietic cells which can specifically regenerate the entire range of red blood cells. At the time of this writing, a handful of people have apparently been cured of SCD in three gene therapy clinical studies with different lentiviral vectors [89].

A number of new sickle cell therapeutic options are on the horizon; the promise of combination therapy is no longer a far-fetched aspiration. This calls for an urgent debate with regards to the correct combinations, the right patient phenotype and access for the majority of patients. It is therefore timely to commission such a review on newborn sickle cell screening not just for European countries which of course face the migration challenge, but also Africa and India [90].

Author Contributions: B.P.D.I. designed the manuscript which was reviewed by L.L.H., W.A., N.K., K.A.A. offering substantial modification and further development of sections. A.P. had written an essay of the role of thrombosis in SCD, some of the concepts were included. K.O.-E. reviewed the manuscript. All authors approved the manuscript.

Funding: This research received no external funding.

Acknowledgments: Temiladeoluwa Bademosi who wrote an essay on a related topic in sickle cell disease as a medical student.

Conflicts of Interest: B.P.D.I. receives educational grant from Global Therapeutics, Pfizer, Novartis plc Cyclerion and honorarium from Novartis plc. L.L.H. is a consultant for Hilton Publishing, Pfizer, AstraZeneca, Emmaus, Emmi Solutions, and University of Cincinnati.

References

1. Herrick, J.B. Peculiar Elongated and Sickle-shaped Red Blood Corpuscles in a Case of Severe Anemiaa. *Yale J. Biol. Med.* **2001**, *74*, 543–548.
2. Hoban, M.D.; Orkin, S.H.; Bauer, D.E. Genetic treatment of a molecular disorder: Gene therapy approaches to sickle cell disease. *Blood* **2016**, *127*, 839–848. [CrossRef] [PubMed]
3. Ingram, V.M. Anecdotal, Historical and Critical Commentaries on Genetics Sickle-Cell Anemia Hemoglobin: The Molecular Biology of the First "Molecular Disease"—The Crucial Importance of Serendipity. *Genetics* **2004**, *167*, 1–7. [CrossRef] [PubMed]
4. Ballas, S.K.; Kesen, M.R.; Goldberg, M.F.; Lutty, G.A.; Dampier, C.; Osunkwo, I.; Wang, W.C.; Hoppe, C.; Hagar, W.; Darbari, D.S.; et al. Beyond the Definitions of the Phenotypic Complications of Sickle Cell Disease: An Update on Management. *Sci. World J.* **2012**, *2012*, 949535. [CrossRef]
5. Weatherall, D.J. The inherited diseases of hemoglobin are an emerging global health burden. *Blood* **2010**, *115*, 4331–4336. [CrossRef] [PubMed]
6. American Society of Haematology. Sickle Cell Disease Family Fact Sheet 2015. Available online: http://www.michigan.gov/documents/mdch/Sickle_Cell_Fact_Sheet_465285_7.pdf (accessed on 10 February 2019).
7. Ansong, D.; Akoto, A.O.; Ocloo, D.; Ohene-frempong, K. Sickle Cell Disease: Management Options and Challenges in Developing Countries. *Mediterr. J. Hematol. Infect. Dis.* **2013**, *5*, e2013062. [CrossRef] [PubMed]
8. Piel, F.B.; Steinberg, M.H.; Rees, D.C. Sickle Cell Disease. *N. Engl. J. Med.* **2017**, *376*, 1561–1573. [CrossRef]
9. Steinberg, M.H. Genetic etiologies for phenotypic diversity in sickle cell anemia. *Sci. World J.* **2009**, *9*, 46–67. [CrossRef]
10. De Montalembert, M. Management of children with sickle cell anemia: A collaborative work. *Arch. Pediatr.* **2002**, *9*, 1195–1201. [PubMed]
11. Weatherall, D.J. The challenge of haemoglobinopathies in resource-poor countries. *Br. J. Haematol.* **2011**, *154*, 736–744. [CrossRef]
12. Grosse, S.D.; Odame, I.; Atrash, H.K.; Amendah, D.D.; Piel, F.B.; Williams, T.N. Sickle cell disease in Africa: A neglected cause of early childhood mortality. *Am. J. Prev. Med.* **2011**, *41*, S398–S405. [CrossRef] [PubMed]
13. Piel, F.B.; Patil, A.P.; Howes, R.E.; Nyangiri, O.A.; Gething, P.W.; Dewi, M.; Temperley, W.H.; Williams, T.N.; Weatherall, D.J.; Hay, S.I. Global epidemiology of sickle haemoglobin in neonates: A contemporary geostatistical model-based map and population estimates. *Lancet* **2013**, *381*, 142–151. [CrossRef]
14. Cronin, E.K.; Normand, C.; Henthorn, J.S.; Hickman, M.; Davies, S.C. Costing model for neonatal screening and diagnosis of haemoglobinopathies. *Arch. Dis. Child. Fetal Neonatal Ed.* **1998**, *79*, F161–F167. [CrossRef] [PubMed]
15. Martinez, P.A.; Angastiniotis, M.; Eleftheriou, A.; Gulbis, B.; Pereira, M.D.; Petrova-Benedict, R.; Corrons, J.L. Haemoglobinopathies in Europe: Health & migration policy perspectives. *Orphanet J. Rare. Dis.* **2014**, *9*, 97.
16. Modell, B.; Petrou, M.; Layton, M.; Slater, C.; Ward, R.H.; Rodeck, C.; Varnavides, L.; Nicolaides, K.; Gibbons, S.; Fitches, A.; et al. Audit of prenatal diagnosis for haemoglobin disorders in the United Kingdom: The first 20 years. *BMJ* **1997**, *315*, 779–784. [CrossRef]
17. Cela, E.; Bellón, J.M.; de la Cruz, M.; Beléndez, C.; Berrueco, R.; Ruiz, A.; Elorza, I.; Díaz de Heredia, C.; Cervera, A.; Valles, G.; et al. National registry of hemoglobinopathies in Spain (REPHem). *Pediatr. Blood Cancer* **2017**, *64*, e26322. [CrossRef] [PubMed]
18. Huntsman, R.G. Hemoglobinopathies: How big a problem? *Can. Med. Assoc. J.* **1978**, *119*, 675. [PubMed]
19. Inusa, B.P.; Colombatti, R. European migration crises: The role of national hemoglobinopathy registries in improving patient access to care. *Pediatr. Blood Cancer* **2017**, *64*, e26515. [CrossRef] [PubMed]
20. Lindenau, J.D.; Wagner, S.C.; Castro, S.M.; Hutz, M.H. The effects of old and recent migration waves in the distribution of HBB* S globin gene haplotypes. *Genet. Mol. Biol.* **2016**, *39*, 515–523. [CrossRef]

21. Dormandy, E.; James, J.; Inusa, B.; Rees, D. How many people have sickle cell disease in the UK? *J. Public Health* **2017**, *40*, e291–e295. [CrossRef]
22. Lobitz, S.; Telfer, P.; Cela, E.; Allaf, B.; Angastiniotis, M.; Backman Johansson, C.; Badens, C.; Bento, C.; Bouva, M.J.; Canatan, D.; et al. Newborn screening for sickle cell disease in Europe: Recommendations from a Pan-European Consensus Conference. *Br. J. Haematol.* **2018**, *183*, 648–660. [CrossRef] [PubMed]
23. Grosse, R.; Lukacs, Z.; Cobos, P.N.; Oyen, F.; Ehmen, C.; Muntau, B.; Timmann, C.; Noack, B. The prevalence of sickle cell disease and its implication for newborn screening in Germany (Hamburg metropolitan area). *Pediatr. Blood Cancer* **2016**, *63*, 168–170. [CrossRef] [PubMed]
24. Colombatti, R.; Martella, M.; Cattaneo, L.; Viola, G.; Cappellari, A.; Bergamo, C.; Azzena, S.; Schiavon, S.; Baraldi, E.; Dalla Barba, B.; et al. Results of a multicenter universal newborn screening program for sickle cell disease in Italy: A call to action. *Pediatr. Blood Cancer* **2019**, *66*, e27657. [CrossRef] [PubMed]
25. Telfer, P.; Coen, P.; Chakravorty, S.; Wilkey, O.; Evans, J.; Newell, H.; Smalling, B.; Amos, R.; Stephens, A.; Rogers, D.; et al. Clinical outcomes in children with sickle cell disease living in England: A neonatal cohort in East London. *haematologica* **2007**, *92*, 905–912. [CrossRef] [PubMed]
26. Quinn, C.T.; Rogers, Z.R.; McCavit, T.L.; Buchanan, G.R. Improved survival of children and adolescents with sickle cell disease. *Blood* **2010**, *115*, 3447–3452. [CrossRef]
27. Makani, J.; Cox, S.E.; Soka, D.; Komba, A.N.; Oruo, J.; Mwamtemi, H.; Magesa, P.; Rwezaula, S.; Meda, E.; Mgaya, J.; et al. Mortality in sickle cell anemia in Africa: A prospective cohort study in Tanzania. *PLoS ONE* **2011**, *6*, e14699. [CrossRef]
28. Chakravorty, S.; Williams, T.N. Sickle cell disease: A neglected chronic disease of increasing global health importance. *Arch. Dis. Child.* **2015**, *100*, 48–53. [CrossRef]
29. Kuznik, A.; Habib, A.G.; Munube, D.; Lamorde, M. Newborn screening and prophylactic interventions for sickle cell disease in 47 countries in sub-Saharan Africa: A cost-effectiveness analysis. *BMC Health Serv. Res.* **2016**, *16*, 304. [CrossRef]
30. Makani, J.; Soka, D.; Rwezaula, S.; Krag, M.; Mghamba, J.; Ramaiya, K.; Cox, S.E.; Grosse, S.D. Health policy for sickle cell disease in Africa: Experience from Tanzania on interventions to reduce under-five mortality. *Trop. Med. Int. Health* **2015**, *20*, 184–187. [CrossRef] [PubMed]
31. Gardner, R.V. Sickle Cell Disease: Advances in Treatment. *Ochsner J.* **2018**, *18*, 377–389. [CrossRef]
32. Manwani, D.; Frenette, P.S. Vaso-occlusion in sickle cell disease: Pathophysiology and novel targeted therapies. *Blood* **2013**, *122*, 3892–3898. [CrossRef] [PubMed]
33. Hebbel, R.P. Ischemia-reperfusion injury in sickle cell anemia: Relationship to acute chest syndrome, endothelial dysfunction, arterial vasculopathy, and inflammatory pain. *Hematol. Oncol. Clin. North Am.* **2014**, *28*, 181–198. [CrossRef]
34. Sebastiani, P.; Nolan, V.G.; Baldwin, C.T.; Abad-Grau, M.M.; Wang, L.; Adewoye, A.H.; McMahon, L.C.; Farrer, L.A.; Taylor, J.G.; Kato, G.J.; et al. A network model to predict the risk of death in sickle cell disease. *Blood* **2007**, *110*, 2727–2735. [CrossRef]
35. Frenette, P.S.; Atweh, G.F. Sickle cell disease: Old discoveries, new concepts, and future promise. *J. Clin. Investig.* **2007**, *117*, 850–858. [CrossRef]
36. Akinsheye, I.; Alsultan, A.; Solovieff, N.; Ngo, D.; Baldwin, C.T.; Sebastiani, P.; Chui, D.H.; Steinberg, M.H. Fetal hemoglobin in sickle cell anemia. *Blood* **2011**, *118*, 19–27. [CrossRef]
37. Bhatnagar, P.; Purvis, S.; Barron-Casella, E.; DeBaun, M.R.; Casella, J.F.; Arking, D.E.; Keefer, J.R. Genome-wide association study identifies genetic variants influencing F-cell levels in sickle-cell patients. *Eur. J. Hum. Genet.* **2011**, *56*, 316. [CrossRef]
38. Watson, J. A study of sickling of young erythrocytes in sickle cell anemia. *Blood* **1948**, *3*, 465–469.
39. Inati, A. Recent advances in improving the management of sickle cell disease. *Blood Rev.* **2009**, *23*, S9–S13. [CrossRef]
40. Bonds, D.R. Three decades of innovation in the management of sickle cell disease: The road to understanding the sickle cell disease clinical phenotype. *Blood Rev.* **2005**, *19*, 99–110. [CrossRef]
41. Watson, R.J.; Burko, H.; Megas, H.; Robinson, M. The hand-foot syndrome in sickle-cell disease in young children. *Pediatrics* **1963**, *31*, 975–982.
42. Piel, F.B.; Tewari, S.; Brousse, V.; Analitis, A.; Font, A.; Menzel, S.; Chakravorty, S.; Thein, S.L.; Inusa, B.; Telfer, P.; et al. Associations between environmental factors and hospital admissions for sickle cell disease. *Haematologica* **2017**, *102*, 666–675. [CrossRef]

43. Brousse, V.; Buffet, P.; Rees, D. The spleen and sickle cell disease: The sick (led) spleen. *Br. J. Haematol.* **2014**, *166*, 165–176. [CrossRef]
44. Minhas, P.S.; KVirdi, J.; Patel, R. Double whammy-acute splenic sequestration crisis in patient with aplastic crisis due to acute parvovirus infection. *J. Commun. Hosp. Int. Med. Perspect.* **2017**, *7*, 194–195. [CrossRef] [PubMed]
45. Tubman, V.N.; Makani, J. Turf wars: Exploring splenomegaly in sickle cell disease in malaria-endemic regions. *Br. J. Haematol.* **2017**, *177*, 938–946. [CrossRef] [PubMed]
46. Booth, C.; Inusa, B.; Obaro, S.K. Infection in sickle cell disease: A review. *Int. J. Infect. Dis.* **2010**, *14*, e2–e12. [CrossRef] [PubMed]
47. Morrissey, B.J.; Bycroft, T.P.; Almossawi, O.; Wilkey, O.B.; Daniels, J.G. Incidence and predictors of bacterial infection in febrile children with sickle cell disease. *Hemoglobin* **2015**, *39*, 316–319. [PubMed]
48. Rezende, P.V.; Viana, M.B.; Murao, M.; Chaves, A.C.; Ribeiro, A.C. Acute splenic sequestration in a cohort of children with sickle cell anemia. *J. Pediatr. (Rio J.)* **2009**, *85*, 163–169. [CrossRef]
49. Araujo, A.N. Acute splenic sequestration in children with sickle cell anemia. *J. Pediatr. (Rio J.)* **2009**, *85*, 373–374. [CrossRef]
50. Habara, A.; Steinberg, M.H. Minireview: Genetic basis of heterogeneity and severity in sickle cell disease. *Exp. Biol. Med.* **2016**, *241*, 689–696. [CrossRef]
51. National Heart Lung and Blood Institute. Evidence-Based Management of Sickle Cell Disease: Expert Panel Report. 2014. Available online: https://www.nhlbi.nih.gov/health-topics/evidence-based-management-sickle-cell-disease (accessed on 10 February 2019).
52. Oteng-Ntim, E.; Meeks, D.; Seed, P.T.; Webster, L.; Howard, J.; Doyle, P.; Chappell, L.C. Adverse maternal and perinatal outcomes in pregnant women with sickle cell disease: Systematic review and meta-analysis. *Blood* **2015**, *125*, 3316–3325. [CrossRef]
53. Anie, K.A.; Green, J. Psychological therapies for sickle cell disease and pain. *Cochrane Database Syst. Rev.* 2015. [CrossRef]
54. Mulder, N.; Nembaware, V.; Adekile, A.; Anie, K.A.; Inusa, B.; Brown, B.; Campbell, A.; Chinenere, F.; Chunda-Liyoka, C.; Derebail, V.K.; et al. Proceedings of a Sickle Cell Disease Ontology workshop—Towards the first comprehensive ontology for sickle cell disease. *Appl. Transl. Genom.* **2016**, *9*, 23–29. [CrossRef]
55. Hsu, L.L.; Green, N.S.; Ivy, E.D.; Neunert, C.E.; Smaldone, A.; Johnson, S.; Castillo, S.; Castillo, A.; Thompson, T.; Hampton, K.; et al. Community health workers as support for sickle cell care. *Am. J. Prev. Med.* **2016**, *51*, S87–S98. [CrossRef]
56. Ohaeri, J.U.; Shokunbi, W.A. Psychosocial burden of sickle cell disease on caregivers in a Nigerian setting. *J. Natl. Med. Assoc.* **2002**, *94*, 1058. [PubMed]
57. Sickle Cell Society. Standards for the Clinical Care of Adults with Sickle Cell Disease in the UK—2018. Available online: https://www.sicklecellsociety.org/sicklecellstandards/ (accessed on 10 Fbruary 2019).
58. Dampier, C.; LeBeau, P.; Rhee, S.; Lieff, S.; Kesler, K.; Ballas, S.; Rogers, Z.; Wang, W.; Comprehensive Sickle Cell Centers (CSCC) Clinical Trial Consortium (CTC) Site Investigators. Health-related quality of life in adults with sickle cell disease (SCD): A report from the comprehensive sickle cell centers clinical trial consortium. *Am. J. Hematol.* **2011**, *86*, 203–205. [CrossRef] [PubMed]
59. Lebensburger, J.D.; Miller, S.T.; Howard, T.H.; Casella, J.F.; Brown, R.C.; Lu, M.; Iyer, R.V.; Sarnaik, S.; Rogers, Z.R.; Wang, W.C.; et al. Influence of severity of anemia on clinical findings in infants with sickle cell anemia: Analyses from the BABY HUG study. *Pediatr. Blood Cancer* **2012**, *59*, 675–678. [CrossRef] [PubMed]
60. Vichinsky, E.P. Comprehensive care in sickle cell disease: Its impact on morbidity and mortality. *Semin. Hematol.* **1991**, *28*, 220–226.
61. Matthews, C.; Walton, E.K.; Inusa, B. Sickle cell disease in childhood. *Stud. BMJ* **2014**, *22*. [CrossRef]
62. Murad, M.H.; Hazem, A.; Prokop, L. Hydroxyurea for Sickle Cell Disease: A Systematic Review of Benefits, Harms, and Barriers of Utilization, 2012 Prepared for the National Heart, Lung, and Blood Institute (NHLBI) Prepared by the Knowledge and Encounter Research Unit. *Mayo Clin.* **2012**, *2012*, 1–116.
63. Ware, R.E. Optimizing hydroxyurea therapy for sickle cell anemia. *ASH Educ. Program Book* **2015**, *2015*, 436–443. [CrossRef]
64. Steinberg, M.H.; Barton, F.; Castro, O.; Pegelow, C.H.; Ballas, S.K.; Kutlar, A.; Orringer, E.; Bellevue, R.; Olivieri, N.; Eckman, J.; et al. Effect of hydroxyurea on mortality and morbidity in adult sickle cell anemia: Risks and benefits up to 9 years of treatment. *JAMA* **2003**, *289*, 1645–1651. [CrossRef] [PubMed]

65. Strouse, J.J.; Lanzkron, S.; Beach, M.C.; Haywood, C.; Park, H.; Witkop, C.; Wilson, R.F.; Bass, E.B.; Segal, J.B. Hydroxyurea for sickle cell disease: A systematic review for efficacy and toxicity in children. *Pediatrics* **2008**, *122*, 1332–1342. [CrossRef] [PubMed]
66. Inusa, B.P.D.; Atoyebi Wale, A.A.; Idhate, T.; Dogara, L.; Ijei, I.; Qin, Y.; Anie, K.; Lawson, J.O.; Hsu, L. Low-dose hydroxycarbamide therapy may offer similar benefit as maximum tolerated dose for children and young adults with sickle cell disease in low-middle-income settings. *F1000Research* **2018**, *7*, F1000 Faculty Rev-1407. [CrossRef]
67. Qureshi, A.; Kaya, B.; Pancham, S.; Keenan, R.; Anderson, J.; Akanni, M.; Howard, J.; British Society for Haematology. Guidelines for the use of hydroxycarbamide in children and adults with sickle cell disease: A British Society for Haematology Guideline. *Br. J. Haematol.* **2018**, *181*, 460–475. [CrossRef]
68. Hassan, A.; Awwalu, S.; Okpetu, L.; Waziri, A.D. Effect of hydroxyurea on clinical and laboratory parameters of sickle cell anaemia patients in North–West Nigeria. *Egypt J. Haematol.* **2017**, *42*, 70. [CrossRef]
69. Niihara, Y.; Miller, S.T.; Kanter, J.; Lanzkron, S.; Smith, W.R.; Hsu, L.L.; Gordeuk, V.R.; Viswanathan, K.; Sarnaik, S.; Osunkwo, I.; Guillaume, E. A phase 3 trial of L-glutamine in sickle cell disease. *N. Engl. J. Med.* **2018**, *379*, 226–235. [CrossRef]
70. Quinn, C.T. L-glutamine for sickle cell anemia: More questions than answers. *Blood* **2018**, *132*, 689–693. [CrossRef]
71. Danaee, A.; Inusa, B.; Howard, J.; Kesse-Adu, R.; Robinson, S. hyperhaemolysis in patients with haemoglobinopathies: A single centre experience: 229. *Br. J. Haematol.* **2014**, *165*, 96.
72. Adewoyin, A.S.; Obieche, J.C. Hypertransfusion therapy in sickle cell disease in Nigeria. *Adv. Hematol.* **2014**, *2014*, 923593. [CrossRef]
73. Kassim, A.A.; Sharma, D. Hematopoietic stem cell transplantation for sickle cell disease: The changing landscape. *Hematol. Oncol. Stem Cell Ther.* **2017**, *10*, 259–266. [CrossRef]
74. Wiebking, V.; Hütker, S.; Schmid, I.; Immler, S.; Feuchtinger, T.; Albert, M.H. Reduced toxicity, myeloablative HLA-haploidentical hematopoietic stem cell transplantation with post-transplantation cyclophosphamide for sickle cell disease. *Ann. Hematol.* **2017**, *96*, 1373–1377. [CrossRef] [PubMed]
75. Hashmi, S.K.; Srivastava, A.; Rasheed, W.; Adil, S.; Wu, T.; Jagasia, M.; Nassar, A.; Hwang, W.Y.; Hamidieh, A.A.; Greinix, H.T.; et al. Cost and quality issues in establishing hematopoietic cell transplant program in developing countries. *Hematol. Oncol. Stem Cell Ther.* **2017**, *10*, 167–172. [CrossRef]
76. Metcalf, B.; Chuang, C.; Dufu, K.; Patel, M.P.; Silva-Garcia, A.; Johnson, C.; Lu, Q.; Partridge, J.R.; Patskovska, L.; Patskovsky, Y.; et al. Discovery of GBT440, an orally bioavailable R-state stabilizer of sickle cell hemoglobin. *ACS Med. Chem. Lett.* **2017**, *8*, 321–326. [CrossRef] [PubMed]
77. Daak, A.A.; Ghebremeskel, K.; Hassan, Z.; Attallah, B.; Azan, H.H.; Elbashir, M.I.; Crawford, M. Effect of omega-3 (n−3) fatty acid supplementation in patients with sickle cell anemia: Randomized, double-blind, placebo-controlled trial. *Am. J. Clin. Nutr.* **2012**, *97*, 37–44. [CrossRef] [PubMed]
78. Tomer, A.; Kasey, S.; Connor, W.E.; Clark, S.; Harker, L.A.; Eckman, J.R. Reduction of pain episodes and prothrombotic activity in sickle cell disease by dietary n-3 fatty acids. *Thromb. Haemost.* **2001**, *85*, 966–974. [CrossRef]
79. Dixit, R.; Nettem, S.; Madan, S.S.; Soe, H.H.; Abas, A.B.; Vance, L.D.; Stover, P.J. Folate supplementation in people with sickle cell disease. *Cochrane. Database Syst. Rev.* 2018. [CrossRef]
80. Adzu, B.; Masimirembwa, C.; Mustapha, K.B.; Thelingwani, R.; Kirim, R.A.; Gamaniel, K.S. Effect of NIPRISAN® on CYP3A4 activity in vitro. *Eur. J. Drug Metab. Pharmacokinet.* **2015**, *40*, 115–118. [CrossRef]
81. Cordeiro, N.J.; Oniyangi, O. Phytomedicines (medicines derived from plants) for sickle cell disease. *Cochrane Database Syst. Rev.* 2004. [CrossRef]
82. Ataga, K.I.; Kutlar, A.; Kanter, J.; Liles, D.; Cancado, R.; Friedrisch, J.; Guthrie, T.H.; Knight-Madden, J.; Alvarez, O.A.; Gordeuk, V.R.; et al. Crizanlizumab for the prevention of pain crises in sickle cell disease. *N. Engl. J. Med.* **2017**, *376*, 429–439. [CrossRef]
83. Kelley, D.; Jones, L.T.; Wu, J.; Bohm, N. Evaluating the safety and effectiveness of venous thromboembolism prophylaxis in patients with sickle cell disease. *J. Thromb. Thrombolysis* **2017**, *43*, 463–468. [CrossRef]
84. Van Zuuren, E.J.; Fedorowicz, Z. Low-molecular-weight heparins for managing vasoocclusive crises in people with sickle cell disease: A summary of a cochrane systematic review. *Hemoglobin* **2014**, *38*, 221–223. [CrossRef]

85. Heeney, M.M.; Hoppe, C.C.; Abboud, M.R.; Inusa, B.; Kanter, J.; Ogutu, B.; Brown, P.B.; Heath, L.E.; Jakubowski, J.A.; Zhou, C.; et al. A multinational trial of prasugrel for sickle cell vaso-occlusive events. *N. Engl. J. Med.* **2016**, *374*, 625–635. [CrossRef]
86. Hoppe, C.C.; Styles, L.; Heath, L.E.; Zhou, C.; Jakubowski, J.A.; Winters, K.J.; Brown, P.B.; Rees, D.C.; Heeney, M.M. Design of the DOVE (Determining Effects of Platelet Inhibition on Vaso-Occlusive Events) trial: A global Phase 3 double-blind, randomized, placebo-controlled, multicenter study of the efficacy and safety of prasugrel in pediatric patients with sickle cell anemia utilizing a dose titration strategy. *Pediatr. Blood Cancer* **2016**, *63*, 299–305.
87. Telen, M.J. Beyond hydroxyurea: New and old drugs in the pipeline for sickle cell disease. *Blood* **2016**, *127*, 810–819. [CrossRef] [PubMed]
88. Zhang, D.; Xu, C.; Manwani, D.; Frenette, P.S. Neutrophils, platelets, and inflammatory pathways at the nexus of sickle cell disease pathophysiology. *Blood* **2016**, *127*, 801–809. [CrossRef] [PubMed]
89. Ribeil, J.A.; Hacein-Bey-Abina, S.; Payen, E.; Magnani, A.; Semeraro, M.; Magrin, E.; Caccavelli, L.; Neven, B.; Bourget, P.; El Nemer, W.; et al. Gene therapy in a patient with sickle cell disease. *N. Engl. J. Med.* **2017**, *376*, 848–855. [CrossRef]
90. Inusa, B.P.; Anie, K.A.; Lamont, A.; Dogara, L.G.; Ojo, B.; Ijei, I.; Atoyebi, W.; Gwani, L.; Gani, E.; Hsu, L. Utilising the 'Getting to Outcomes®' Framework in Community Engagement for Development and Implementation of Sickle Cell Disease Newborn Screening in Kaduna State, Nigeria. *Int. J. Neonatal Screen.* **2018**, *4*, 33. [CrossRef]

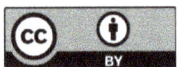

© 2019 by the authors. Licensee MDPI, Basel, Switzerland. This article is an open access article distributed under the terms and conditions of the Creative Commons Attribution (CC BY) license (http://creativecommons.org/licenses/by/4.0/).

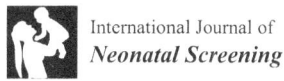 International Journal of
Neonatal Screening

Review

Thalassemias: An Overview

Michael Angastiniotis [1],* and Stephan Lobitz [2]

1 Thalassemia International Federation, Strovolos 2083, Nicosia, Cyprus
2 Department of Pediatric Oncology/Hematology, Kinderkrankenhaus Amsterdamer Straße, 50735 Cologne, Germany; LobitzS@Kliniken-Koeln.de
* Correspondence: michael.angastiniotis@thalassaemia.org.cy; Tel.: +357-22-319129

Received: 2 November 2018; Accepted: 18 March 2019; Published: 20 March 2019

Abstract: Thalassemia syndromes are among the most serious and common genetic conditions. They are indigenous in a wide but specific geographical area. However, through migration they are spreading across regions not previously affected. Thalassemias are caused by mutations in the α (*HBA1/HBA2*) and β globin (*HBB*) genes and are usually inherited in an autosomal recessive manner. The corresponding proteins form the adult hemoglobin molecule (HbA) which is a heterotetramer of two α and two β globin chains. Thalassemia-causing mutations lead to an imbalanced globin chain production and consecutively to impaired erythropoiesis. The severity of the disease is largely determined by the degree of chain imbalance. In the worst case, survival is dependent on regular blood transfusions, which in turn cause transfusional iron overload and secondary multi-organ damage due to iron toxicity. A vigorous monitoring and treatment regime is required, even for the milder syndromes. Thalassemias are a major public health issue in many populations which many health authorities fail to address. Even though comprehensive care has resulted in long-term survival and good quality of life, poor access to essential components of management results in complications which increase the cost of treatment and lead to poor outcomes. These requirements are not recognized by measures such as the Global Burden of Disease project, which ranks thalassemia very low in terms of disability-adjusted life years (DALYs), and fails to consider that it ranks highly in the one to four-year-old age group, making it an important contributor to under-5 mortality. Thalassemia does not fulfil the criteria to be accepted as a target disease for neonatal screening. Nevertheless, depending on the screening methodology, severe cases of thalassemia will be detected in most neonatal screening programs for sickle cell disease. This is very valuable because: (1) it helps to prepare the affected families for having a sick child and (2) it is an important measure of secondary prevention.

Keywords: thalassemia; burden of disease; newborn screening; hemoglobinopathies

1. Introduction

The hereditary disorders of the hemoglobin molecule are among the commonest of clinically serious genetic conditions [1]. They are of two general types: those in which a mutation interferes with the amount of protein produced (thalassemias), and those that result in a structural change of the hemoglobin molecule, leading to the production of a variant protein (hemoglobinopathies).

In this article we will review the pathophysiology and the clinical and public health consequences of thalassemias. These include two categories, the α- and β-thalassemias, according to which the globin chain of the hemoglobin molecule is inadequately produced. The clinically most serious conditions are the β-thalassemias in the homozygous state, while the α-thalassemia homozygotes are usually lethal in utero.

The numbers of affected patients are not known. Very few countries maintain a patient registry and in many others, children die from the more severe transfusion-dependent syndromes before they are even diagnosed. Rough estimates of expected global annual births are around

60,000 [1]. The distribution of the thalassemia genes stretches from the Mediterranean basin and Sub-Saharan Africa through the Middle East to the Far East including South China and the Pacific Islands. In northern regions, these genes are rare in the indigenous populations, but population movements, both for economic reasons and due to political instability, are contributing to a changing epidemiology [2,3]. The necessity for lifelong treatment, the prevention of serious complications through regular monitoring, and premature deaths in many patients make these disorders a significant health burden requiring public health planning and policy making [4]. This is a process which countries with few resources are often unable to follow. Even in the well-resourced countries of the West, the rarity of the condition does not always allow for expertise to develop, and optimum care is also lacking here.

2. Pathophysiology of Thalassemias

In the physiological state, the hemoglobin molecule is a heterotetramer consisting of two α and two non-α globin chains, each carrying a heme molecule with a central iron. In this state, the oxygen-carrying capacity of the molecule is maximal. The non-α globin chains can be β chains which coupled with α chains form adult hemoglobin (HbA), while α chains and δ chains form a minor fraction of adult hemoglobin (HbA$_2$). Finally, α and γ chains form the fetal hemoglobin (HbF). The production of the globin chains is regulated by the α globin cluster on chromosome 16 with the two α globin genes *HBA1* and *HBA2*, and the β globin cluster on chromosome 11 with the genes for the γ, δ, and β globin chains. The physiological situation is characterized by a balanced production of the α and the non-α globin chains that ensures a reciprocal pairing into the normal tetramers. In the thalassemias, this equilibrium is disrupted by the defective production of one of the globin chains. Any reduced production of one of the globin chains within the developing red cell will cause an accumulation of the normally produced chain that can no longer find the equivalent amount of its heterologous partner to assemble to the normal heterotetramer. If α globin chains are not produced in adequate amounts there will be an accumulation of β globin chains (α-thalassemia); if β globin chains are inadequately produced then α globin chains will accumulate (β-thalassemia). These observations were made possible by the introduction of methods to separate and quantify these globin chains [5,6]. These studies enabled the understanding of the pathophysiology of these conditions as being the result of the chain imbalance [7].

The excess unpaired and insoluble α globin chains in β-thalassemia cause apoptosis of red cell precursors, resulting in ineffective erythropoiesis. The excess non-α globin chains in α-thalassemia assemble as γ$_4$ tetramers (Hb Bart's) in intrauterine life and β$_4$ tetramers (HbH) after birth. Both of these abnormal homotetramers are poor carriers of oxygen (too high affinity for oxygen). The excess chains have further devastating effects on the function of erythrocytes and their ability to deliver oxygen [8,9].

- The production of hemoglobin starts in the proerythroblast and increases during erythroid maturation through the basophilic, polychromatophilic and orthochromatic phases of red cell maturation. In erythroblasts, the excess α globin chains in β-thalassemia precipitate at the cell membrane and cause oxidative membrane damage and premature cell death by apoptosis. This happens within the erythropoietic tissue and so results in ineffective erythropoiesis [10].
- Some of the immature red cells pass into the circulation. Because of their membrane defect, they are fragile and prone to hemolysis. They also exhibit an altered deformability and are trapped by the spleen where they are destroyed by macrophages. This leads to an enlargement of the spleen which can become massive, leading to the development of functional hypersplenism with removal of platelets and white cells as well as red cells.
- Ineffective erythropoiesis, removal of abnormal cells by the spleen, and hemolysis all contribute to an anemia of variable severity.

The response to anemia is twofold:

- The kidneys increase secretion of erythropoietin (EPO). EPO is a cytokine that targets red cell precursors in response to the oxygen requirement of tissues. EPO secretion results in an increased red cell production, but because of the defect of erythroblast maturation this will make the ineffective erythropoiesis worse. This is a vicious cycle that results in expansion of hematopoietic tissue within the bone marrow and the destruction of bone architecture, thus contributing to bone disease and fragility. In some patients, extramedullary hematopoietic masses develop within the liver, the spleen, and the reticuloendothelial system.
- Hepcidin is a regulator of iron absorption [11] and produced by liver cells. It regulates the expression of ferroportin, a protein which directly facilitates enterocytic iron absorption in the gut. Independently of the cause, in severe anemia, hepcidin production is suppressed which results in increased iron absorption [12]. This contributes to iron overload, especially in patients who are not regularly transfused.

The degree of anemia is variable and depends on the mutation or combination of mutations in each individual patient. There are about 200 known mutations on the β gene cluster. Some mutations do not allow any β globin chain production. These are known as $β^0$ mutations while other mutations allow some β globin chain production and are referred to as $β^+$ and $β^{++}$ mutations, respectively [13]. Likewise, in α-thalassemia more than 100 varieties have been described [14]. The degree of anemia and the severity of the clinical effect can be modified by other mitigating factors. The most common of these is the co-inheritance of factors that reduce globin chain imbalance such as when α-thalassemia is co-inherited in β-thalassemia homozygotes, resulting in a milder β-thalassemia syndrome.

The treatment of severe anemia is blood transfusion. In the serious transfusion dependent forms, regular transfusions from early childhood lead to severe iron overload. In the physiological state 1–2 mg of iron are absorbed from food sources daily and the same amount is excreted fecally. Increased gastrointestinal absorption of iron in thalassemia aggravates transfusional iron burden and results in the excess iron being taken up by proteins produced in the liver, including transferrin and ferritin. Protein bound iron is stored mainly in the liver and is not toxic. However, since each unit of transfused blood contains 100–200 mg of iron (0.47 mg/mL), in regularly transfused patients, the capacity of these proteins to bind iron is saturated soon and non-transferrin bound iron (NTBI) is released into the plasma [15,16]. This free iron, particularly a species known as labile plasma iron (LPI), generates reactive-oxygen species resulting in organelle damage and cell death, especially of hepatocytes, cardiomyocytes and the cells of endocrine glands [17]. Vital organ function is disturbed in this way, leading to serious complications which may be lethal. This necessitates the daily consumption of iron chelating agents to prevent complications and ensure survival. The degree to which these effects of iron overload occur is related to transfusion dependency. In non-transfusion dependent forms of thalassemia (NTDT), such as β-thalassemia intermedia and α-thalassemia, there is also iron overload secondary to increased absorption from the gut. However, this develops at a much slower rate than in transfusion-dependent thalassemia (TDT) [18]. Complications in these NTDT appear later in life, mostly in the second and third decades (the clinical effects of NTDT are summarized below).

3. Clinical Considerations

According to the causative genetic defect, the thalassemia syndromes are usually classified as β- or α-thalassemias. Here, in Table 1, we attempt to use a classification according to clinical severity, which may include several genetic types in one category.

Table 1. Thalassemia groupings according to clinical severity.

α-Thalassemia hydrops fetalis	Leads to death in utero in most cases
Transfusion-dependent (β) thalassemia	Leads to death in early infancy unless treated
Non transfusion-dependent thalassemia	Occasional blood transfusions required (may become transfusion-dependent in later life)
Thalassemia minor	Mostly heterozygotes for thalassemia genes (carriers), but may include some homozygotes/compound heterozygotes for very mild β-thalassemia mutations and HbE

Alpha thalassemia hydrops fetalis is caused by deletion or inactivation of all four α globin alleles. The result is that excess gamma globin chains form tetramers (γ_4 = Hb Bart's) in uterine life, which because of their high oxygen affinity cannot effectively deliver oxygen to tissues. This leads to severe hypoxia [19]. Intrauterine anemia leads to heart failure although the underlying mechanisms are still to be fully understood [20]. There are signs of pronounced fetal edema, hepatosplenomegaly and hydramnios. Maternal pre-eclampsia and the need for caesarean section endanger mother's health and life. These possible outcomes have made it a rule that prenatal diagnosis is offered to at-risk pregnancies with termination of pregnancy before maternal health is affected. However, intra-uterine blood transfusions have led some pregnancies to a successful outcome and the babies to survive as transfusion dependent patients [21]. The molecular defects that can cause hydrops include deletional mutations found in the Mediterranean countries like $-^{MED}/-^{MED}$, but more commonly in Asia like $-^{SEA}/-^{SEA}$; in addition, in South East Asia severe non-deletional mutations are more common, and so hydrops is more commonly encountered in that region. Some of these non-deletional mutations correspond to a mixed defect in which the thalassemic determinant is associated with an unstable abnormal hemoglobin. Examples are Constant Spring (common), Quong Sze, Suan Dok, Pakse, and Adana (rare) hemoglobin [22].

TDTs are the most serious clinical entities which become clinically apparent in infancy and result from β^0 or severe β^+ homozygosity. Triplication or quadruplication of α genes aggravate β-thalassemia and can even transform a classically asymptomatic β-thalassemia heterozygosity into a clinically relevant condition.

The hallmark of TDT is a steadily progressive anemia which makes the child transfusion-dependent from the first few months of life. The onset of clinical symptoms coincides with the fetal to adult hemoglobin switch in which HbF production decreases and is normally replaced by the production of HbA. However, because of the thalassemic defect, the switch is either abolished (β^0/β^0 homozygosity) or the production of HbA is grossly insufficient to compensate for the HbF decrease (β^0/β^+ or severe β^+/β^+). The continuous fall of the hemoglobin level and all the consequences described above lead to the need for repeated blood transfusions. The therapeutic aim is to keep a level of hemoglobin that will not only ensure good oxygenation, but also reduce the stimulus for EPO secretion and thus reduce endogenous erythropoiesis [23]. Keeping the pre-transfusion hemoglobin above 9–10 g/dL achieves this aim and allows for physical development with reduced or no bony changes and deformities. Regular lifelong transfusions have several possible adverse effects which include immunological reactions and transmission of infectious agents of which the hepatitis C virus is currently the most common. In many countries, inadequate supplies of donors result in low hemoglobin levels, with the consequences of anemia described before. The most important side effect, however, is the accumulation of iron, the pathophysiological consequences of which have been described above. The life endangering effects of iron toxicity necessitate close monitoring and quantification of the iron load in the tissues and removal of the iron by iron chelating agents [24]. The thalassemia patient is therefore subjected to a series of tests aiming at prevention or at least early recognition of tissue toxicity.

Regular monitoring of regularly transfused patients includes

- Regular blood tests: hematology, biochemistry and serology
- Imaging: MRI (to measure heart and liver iron load), abdominal ultrasound, bone density
- Echocardiography to assess cardiac function and pulmonary hypertension
- Ophthalmological examinations and audiometry
- Organ biopsies as required (largely replaced by MRI)

On a global level, effective iron chelation is hampered by:

- Poor availability of drugs in many countries and catastrophic out of pocket expenses [25].
- Patient non-adherence to prescribed treatment [26]. In many clinics, non-adherence is regarded as a major cause of treatment failure. This is not surprising since chelation treatment is a daily routine, and any short or long interruption leads to the exposure of cells to free iron radicals with consecutive tissue damage. Various interventions have been suggested to reduce this phenomenon mainly relying on psychosocial support and the patient partaking in management decisions which concern them. Understanding patient concerns is still an open subject [27,28] and effective interventions are still a problem in everyday life of thalassemia clinics across the world.
- Inexperience and inadequate adherence of physicians to evidence based guidelines. This is a phenomenon which is not well documented in scientific publications but is a common experience where rare conditions are concerned [29]. Due to the rarity of the condition in many localities, thalassemia suffers from all the weaknesses reported by EURORDIS and other rare disease organizations, such as delayed diagnosis and recognizing life-threatening complications too late [30].

The long survival experienced by the latest birth cohorts of patients with the most severe thalassemia syndromes, mainly treated in centers of expertise, is due to a combination of safe and effective blood transfusion, adequate iron chelation and early recognition of complications with effective interventions by a multidisciplinary team of experts. The excellent outcomes in terms of survival and quality of life were not achieved by the introduction of new additional therapies [31], but by adherence to evidence-based guidelines. New treatments are expected in the near future [32] which will probably further improve quality of life. Curative treatments, apart from haemopoietic stem cell transplantation (HSCT) which has long been available [33], are also in the pipeline, utilizing genetic therapies.

Milder, non-transfusion dependent forms (NTDT), which can survive without regular blood transfusions may require occasional transfusions during intercurrent illnesses or pregnancies. However, regular transfusions may be required in later life due to complications. NTDT syndromes are caused by mild β^{++} mutations (allowing some β globin chain production) and/or the co-inheritance of mitigating factors such as α-thalassemia or persistence of fetal hemoglobin which reduce the globin chain imbalance. Another mechanism is the co-inheritance of another hemoglobin variant, the most common being HbE which is commonly encountered in South East Asia [34]. HbE is a "thalassemic variant", i.e., a hemoglobin variant that is produced insufficiently and thus promotes anemia.

Since erythropoietic tissue expansion is not suppressed early in life by transfusions, its effects on bone marrow expansion and extramedullary erythropoiesis continues and so damage to bone structure, leading to deformities and relatively early onset of osteopenia/osteoporosis and pressure from hematopoietic masses, characterize this syndrome. Chronic anemia and ineffective erythropoiesis persist despite a relatively steady hemoglobin level with the result of increasing iron absorption from the gut through hepcidin suppression. This causes iron toxicity mainly to the liver while the heart remains relatively free of iron-related damage [35–37]. Iron overload with the increased circulation of NTBI leads to hepatocyte damage which progresses to fibrosis, presumably due to longer duration of exposure [38] and to hepatocellular carcinoma, which is more frequent in NTDT. Erythropoietic expansion as evidenced by the respective markers like soluble transferrin receptors (sTfR), increased nucleated red cells (NRBCs) and growth differentiation factor 15 (GDF-15) [39], will also contribute to splenomegaly leading many clinicians to recommend splenectomy. The pathophysiological effects of splenectomy and hypercoagulability are more often encountered in NTDT compared to TDT and so stroke, pulmonary hypertension and vascular disease are more frequent in NTDT compared to regularly transfused patients. It is because of these complications that splenectomy is avoided and that regular transfusions are initiated in NTDT patients when complications arise such as symptomatic extramedullary hematopoietic masses, pulmonary hypertension, thrombotic events, and leg ulcers [40]. Interestingly, causative factors of NTDT are variable, including mostly β-thalassemia intermedia and HbE/β-thalassemia but also HbH disease (which belongs to the α-thalassemia group). There are differences in both the biomarkers of iron metabolism and erythropoiesis as well as in the clinical manifestations among the various causative factors [39]. For instance, HbH disease in the Mediterranean has the mildest effects but can be severe in South East Asia. Similarly, for unknown reasons, HbE/β-thalassemia presentation varies from relatively moderate to very severe.

4. Management of the Thalassemia Syndromes: The Global Perspective

It is not possible here to go over the details of all treatment modalities and their possible effectiveness or side effects. The impression in many high prevalence areas is that providing adequate supplies of 'clean' blood and a choice of iron chelating agents is the basis of managing these syndromes effectively. This is particularly true if the thalassemia population consists of children. From adolescence and even earlier, a monitoring schedule should be in place, aiming to recognize early complications which should be dealt with. Centers, mainly in the economically developed world, which are able to fully follow internationally accepted guidelines [41] are serving a minority of the global community of patients [1,3,4]. Such privileged patients are now surviving to their fifties with a good quality of life. Even in locations with few resources, essential components of care cannot be ignored or put aside because of "other priorities". The reason is that any reductions will increase the chance of complications and so increase the cost of care and/or result in premature death. This is a waste of resources that is often not recognized. The burden of disease, in the case of congenital disorders, cannot be simply assessed by the numbers of patients affected. In the reports of the Global Burden of Disease (GBD), thalassemia was ranked 68th in 2010 in terms of DALYs, yet it ranked 24th when the one-to-four-year age group was considered, indicating its important contribution to under-5 mortality [42]. It is doubtful whether this ranking is based on accurate data since many children in countries with high prevalence of thalassemia and with less privileged populations may die without even a diagnosis. National policies are usually formulated by public health officials who have no clinical experience and use DALYs and GBD data to rank their country's priorities. The hemoglobin disorders are therefore not regarded as a priority. Late-onset diseases such as cardiovascular disorders and diabetes are given high ranking and are prioritized, even by WHO in its non-communicable disease (NCD) program, leaving congenital and hereditary disorders with no plan either for patient survival or even for prevention. The results are disastrous, and early death often makes the problem invisible [4]. Any improvements in thalassemia management will benefit health services for many needs in the community:

- Adequacy of blood supplies—Regularly transfused patients require more blood than the general population and so blood collection drives, donor education, and good practices in donor management are organized. These efforts which aim to have adequate supplies will benefit the whole community and patients who require blood transfusion circumstantially for whatever reason will also benefit
- Safe blood—Regularly transfused patients are at higher risk from contaminated blood from both bacteria and viruses, and in some locations malaria is also a threat. Having strict screening procedures to screen donors will make blood safer for all the community.

- Reactions to blood transfusion are more common in regularly transfused patients, especially alloimmunization. Having procedures and technology for leukodepletion and extended antigen typing (including molecular typing) in place, will help many patients in the community (N.B., regularly transfused patients are not only those with hemoglobin disorders but include other congenital anemias, myelodysplasias, and bleeding disorders).
- Having availability of quality medication, so that effectiveness and safety of drugs is guaranteed, is a universal requirement. As generic drugs are increasingly becoming available and affordable, their quality should be more strictly controlled. This will help all patients, especially those with life-long dependency due to chronic disease.
- Centers of expertise are healthcare facilities where standards of care for chronic and rare diseases can be guaranteed. Coordinated multidisciplinary teams have been shown to improve patient outcomes where multi-organ disorders are concerned [43]. Centers of expertise can support other centers with fewer patients and less experience in an organized and officially recognized networking system. This is a universal recommendation supported by a system of accreditation of centers. This concept has been recognized by the European Commission through projects like EURORDIS and ENERCA which has resulted in criteria for centers of expertise [44,45] and the creation of European Reference Networks (ERNs) for rare diseases including rare anemias. The Thalassemia International Federation (TIF) is now developing disease-specific standards aiming at the accreditation of centers as a means for quality improvement.
- Following evidence-based guidelines is another universal recommendation.

  - Universal health coverage will ensure that families are not bankrupted by the demands of a chronic lifelong condition. Out of pocket expenses are the major reason why in some countries optimum care is not accessible for all patients—with all the known consequences. "Health is a human right. No one should get sick and die just because they are poor, or because they cannot access the health services they need" (Dr. Tedros Adhanom Ghebreyesus, Director General WHO, World Health Day 2018 Advocacy Toolkit; 7th April 2018; https://www.who.int/campaigns/world-health-day/2018/World-Health-Day-2018-Policy-Advocacy-Toolkit-Final.pdf?ua=1; last access: 20 March 2019)

5. Prevention and Screening

Prevention programs have reduced the birth prevalence of thalassemia in some countries and possibly saved resources for patient care. Such programs require planning and investment in order to include public awareness, screening to identify carriers, genetic counselling aiming to assist couples in making informed choices, and finally making available solutions such as prenatal diagnosis [46]. There are considerable differences in the attitude of people towards screening as well as for prenatal diagnosis and termination of pregnancy. Cultural, religious, ethical, and legal considerations must be considered in each country, but also, in this era of increasing population mix, different attitudes within communities in any country have to be considered in planning services [47]. Even though prevention has been shown to be cost-effective [48] very few countries have adopted nationally planned programs.

Neonatal screening to identify thalassemia syndromes early is not of great benefit especially in high prevalence areas where full prevention programs are in effect, since the clinical manifestations and transfusion dependency appear early in life. Where neonatal screening for sickle cell disease is established, some thalassemia homozygote cases and hemoglobin variants can be identified using the same laboratory techniques (mainly high-pressure liquid chromatography [48] and/or capillary electrophoresis and even isoelectric focusing). However, in many countries' patients are not identified and/or there is no patient registry on a national level and so the numbers are not known. In these situations, neonatal screening (when universal) can be useful in collecting more accurate data than surveys which often include small cohorts of a population:

- Hemoglobin variants can be accurately identified and so result in the well-known benefits of screening for sickle cell disease and epidemiological data on other variants can be obtained.
- Epidemiology of α-thalassemia can also be obtained through the detection of Hb Bart's [49].
- Thalassemia major can be identified in neonatal blood by using a cut off value of 1.5% HbA [50,51].

These tests are useful for secondary prevention and epidemiological studies, especially if supplemented by molecular studies. Other forms of technology such as tandem mass spectrometry may even be sensitive enough to identify β-thalassemia heterozygotes [52].

6. Conclusions

The thalassemia syndromes are hereditary disorders with a complex pathophysiology and serious multi-organ involvement. Current treatment may lead to long survival and a good quality of life. This includes benefitting from a full education, marriage, and parenthood, as well as contributing to the society as ordinary citizens do. In contrast, for the majority of patients, access to quality and holistic care is not possible. For these patients, thalassemia is a tragic disease with life-threatening complications which imply death in adolescence or early adulthood and result in a life of disability. Even in well-organized and well-resourced health services the provision of adequate supplies of safe blood and iron chelation are thought to meet patient needs, often ignoring the role of endocrine, cardiac, and liver monitoring by specialized teams which can deal with emerging vital organ dysfunction. The need for at least one expert reference center supporting secondary centers within each country in an organized network must be part of a policy directed and supported at the central level. This is in accordance with the concept of European Reference Networks (ERNs) for rare disorders; thalassemia falls into this category of disease in most countries.

Emerging new therapies, such as genetic interventions aiming to reduce globin chain imbalance, are likely to benefit those able to afford current management modalities leaving the "silent majority" to struggle with what basic treatments that they can afford. The solution is for health authorities to meet their obligations to those born with these conditions and persuade society and economists that investment in their health is meeting an obligation to human rights.

In this picture the question is whether neonatal screening programs can effectively contribute to achieve the desired outcomes. In areas where effective pre-conceptual or premarital prevention programs are fully applied, few cases will be picked up postnatally. In such a setting, new-born affected infants are often in families which have been informed and have chosen to give birth to an affected child. Even where there is no prevention policy, infants generally present clinically at a very young age and require immediate intervention due to severe anemia. To develop a policy solely for the early detection of thalassemia does not seem necessary. However, where there is a program for the detection of sickle cell disease, some thalassemia syndromes and most variants may be identified. This can be beneficial for secondary prevention but also in some settings for the early detection of new cases.

Author Contributions: Conceptualization, M.A.; Writing—Original Draft Preparation, M.A.; Writing—Review & Editing, M.A., S.L.

Funding: This research received no external funding.

Conflicts of Interest: The authors declare no conflict of interest.

References

1. Modell, B.; Darlison, M. Global epidemiology of haemoglobin disorders and derived service indicators. *Bull. World Health Organ.* **2008**, *86*, 480–487. [CrossRef]
2. Angastiniotis, M.; Vives Corrons, J.L.; Soteriades, E.S.; Eleftheriou, A. The impact of migrations on the health services of Europe: The example of haemoglobin disorders. *Sci. World J.* **2013**, *2013*, 727905. [CrossRef] [PubMed]
3. Weatherall, D.J. The inherited diseases of haemoglobin are an emerging global health burden. *Blood* **2010**, *115*, 4331–4333. [CrossRef] [PubMed]

4. Weatherall, D.J. The challenge of haemoglobinopathies in poor resource countries. *Br. J. Haematol.* **2011**, *154*, 736–744. [CrossRef] [PubMed]
5. Clegg, J.B.; Naughton, M.A.; Weatherall, D.J. An improved method for the characterisation of human haemoglobin mutants: Identification of alpha-2-beta-95 GLU haemoglobin N (Baltimore). *Nature* **1965**, *207*, 944. [CrossRef]
6. Weatherall, D.J.; Clegg, J.B.; Naughton, M.A. Globin synthesis in thalassaemia: An in vitro study. *Nature* **1965**, *208*, 1061–1065. [CrossRef] [PubMed]
7. Nathan, D.G.; Gunn, R.B. Thalassemia: The consequence of unbalanced haemoglobin synthesis. *Am. J. Med.* **1966**, *41*, 815–830. [CrossRef]
8. Nathan, D.G.; Strossel, T.B.; Gunn, R.B.; Zarkowsky, H.S.; Laforet, M.T. Influence of haemoglobin precipitation on erythrocyte metabolism in alpha and beta thalassaemia. *J. Clin. Investig.* **1969**, *48*, 33–41. [CrossRef] [PubMed]
9. Nienhuis, A.W.; Nathan, D.G. Pathophysiology and clinical manifestations of the β-thalassemias. *Cod. Spring Harb. Perspect. Med.* **2012**, *2*, a011726. [CrossRef]
10. Rivella, S. Ineffective erythropoiesis and thalassemias. *Curr. Opin. Hematol.* **2009**, *16*, 187–194. [CrossRef]
11. Ganz, T. Hepcidin, a key regulator of iron metabolism and mediator of anemia of inflammation. *Blood* **2003**, *102*, 783–788. [CrossRef]
12. Papanikolaou, G.; Tzilianos, M.; Christakis, J.I.; Bagdanos, D.; Tsimirika, K.; MacFarlane, J.; Goldberg, Y.P.; Sakellaropoulos, N.; Ganz, T.; Nemeth, E. Hepcidin in iron overload disorders. *Blood* **2005**, *105*, 4103–4105. [CrossRef]
13. Higgs, D.R.; Engel, J.D.; Stamatoyannopoulos, G. Thalassaemia. *Lancet* **2012**, *379*, 373–383. [CrossRef]
14. Piel, F.; Weatherall, D.J. The alpha thalassaemias. *N. Engl. J. Med.* **2014**, *371*, 1908–1916. [CrossRef]
15. Porter, J.B. Practical management of iron overload. *Br. J. Haematol.* **2001**, *115*, 239–252. [CrossRef]
16. Porter, J.B.; Garbowski, M. The pathophysiology of transfusion iron overload. *Hematol. Oncol. Clin. N. Am.* **2014**, *28*, 683. [CrossRef]
17. Fibach, E.; Rachmilevitz, E. The role of anti-oxidants and iron chelators in the treatment of oxidative stress in thalassaemia. *Ann. N. Y. Acad. Sci.* **2010**, *1202*, 10–16. [CrossRef]
18. Taher, A.; Weatherall, D.J.; Cappellini, M.D. Thalassaemia. *Lancet* **2018**, *391*, 115–167. [CrossRef]
19. Origa, R.; Moi, P. Alpha thalassaemia. In *GeneReviews®[Internet]*; Adam, M.P., Ardinger, H.H., Pagon, R.A., Wallace, S.E., Bean, L.J.H., Stephens, K., Amemiya, A., Eds.; University of Washington, Seattle: Seattle, WA, USA, 2005.
20. Jatavan, P.; Chattipakorn, N.; Tongsong, T. Fetal haemoglobin Bart's hydrops fetalis: Pathophysiology, prenatal diagnosis and possibility of intrauterine treatment. *J. Mater. Fetal. Neonatal. Med.* **2018**, *31*, 946–957. [CrossRef]
21. Songdej, D.; Babbs, C.; Higgs, D.R.; BHFS Consortium. An international registry of survivors with haemoglobin Bart's hydrops fetalis syndrome. *Blood* **2017**, *129*, 1251–1259. [CrossRef]
22. Farashi, S.; Harteveld, C.L. Molecular basis of α-thalassaemia. *Blood Cells Mol. Dis.* **2018**, *70*, 43–53. [CrossRef] [PubMed]
23. Cazzola, M.; De Stefano, P.; Ponchio, L.; Locatelli, F.; Beguin, Y.; Dessi, C.; Barella, S.; Cao, A.; Galanello, R. Relationship between transfusion regimen and suppression of erythropoiesis in beta-thalassaemia major. *Br. J. Haematol.* **1995**, *89*, 473–478. [CrossRef] [PubMed]
24. Porter, J.B.; Garbowski, M.W. Interaction of transfusion and iron chelation in thalassaemia. *Hematol. Oncol. Clin. N. Am.* **2018**, *32*, 247–259. [CrossRef]
25. Hisam, A.; Sadiq Khan, N.; Tariq, N.A.; Irfan, H.; Arif, B.; Noor, M. Perceived stress and monetary burden among thalassaemia patients and their caregivers. *Pak. J. Med. Sci.* **2018**, *34*, 901–906. [CrossRef]
26. Fortin, P.M.; Fisher, S.A.; Madgwick, K.V.; Trivella, M.; Hopewell, S.; Doree, C.; Estcourt, L.J. Strategies to increase adherence to iron chelation therapy in people with sickle cell disease or thalassaemia. *Cochrane Database Syst. Rev.* **2018**. [CrossRef] [PubMed]
27. Trachtenberg, F.L.; Mednick, L.; Kwiatkowski, J.L.; Neufeld, E.J.; Haines, D.; Pakbaz, Z.; Thompson, A.A.; Quinn, C.T.; Grady, R.; Sobota, A.; et al. Beliefs about chelation among thalassemia patients. *Health Qual. Life Outcomes* **2012**, *10*, 148. [CrossRef] [PubMed]
28. Vosper, J.; Evangeli, M.; Porter, J.B.; Shah, F. Psychological factors associated with episodic chelation adherence in thalassaemia. *Hemoglobin* **2018**, *42*, 30–36. [CrossRef] [PubMed]

29. Budych, K.; Helms, T.M.; Schultz, C. How do patients with rare diseases experience the medical encounter? Exploring role behaviour and the impact on patient physician interaction. *Health Policy* **2012**, *105*, 154–164. [CrossRef]
30. EURORDIS. Rare Disease: Understanding the Public Health Policy. 2005. Available online: www.eurordis.org (accessed on 20 March 2019).
31. Taher, A.T.; Cappellini, M.D. How I manage medical complications of beta thalassemia in adults. *Blood* **2018**, *132*, 1781–1791. [CrossRef] [PubMed]
32. Cappellini, M.D.; Porter, J.B.; Viprakasit, V.; Taher, A.T. A paradigm shift on beta thalassaemia treatment: How will we manage this old disease with new therapies? *Blood Rev.* **2018**, *32*, 300–311. [CrossRef]
33. Shenoy, S.; Angelucci, E.; Arnold, S.D.; Baker, K.S.; Bhatia, M.; Bresters, D.; Dietz, A.C.; De La Fuente, J.; Duncan, C.; Gaziev, J.; et al. Current Results and Future Research Priorities in Late Effects after Hematopoietic Stem Cell Transplantation for Children with Sickle Cell Disease and Thalassemia: A Consensus Statement from the Second Pediatric Blood and Marrow Transplant Consortium International Conference on Late Effects after Pediatric Hematopoietic Stem Cell Transplantation. *Biol. Blood Marrow. Transplant.* **2017**, *23*, 552–561. [PubMed]
34. Sleiman, J.; Tarhini, A.; Bou-Fakhredin, R.; Saliba, A.N.; Cappellini, M.D.; Taher, A.T. Non-Transfusion-Dependent Thalassemia: An Update on Complications and Management. *Int. J. Mol. Sci.* **2018**, *19*, 182. [CrossRef] [PubMed]
35. Bou-Fakhredin, R.; Bazarbachi, A.H.; Chaya, B.; Sleiman, J.; Cappellini, M.D.; Taher, A.T. Iron Overload and Chelation Therapy in Non-Transfusion Dependent Thalassemia. *Int. J. Mol. Sci.* **2017**, *18*, 2778. [CrossRef] [PubMed]
36. Mavrogeni, S.; Gotsis, E.; Ladis, V.; Berdousis, E.; Verganelakis, D.; Toulas, P.; Cokkinos, D.V. Magnetic resonance evaluation of liver and myocardial iron deposition in thalassemia intermedia and b-thalassemia major. *Int. J. Cardiovasc. Imaging* **2008**, *24*, 849–854. [CrossRef] [PubMed]
37. Origa, R.; Barella, S.; Argiolas, G.M.; Bina, P.; Agus, A.; Galanello, R. No evidence of cardiac iron in 20 never- or minimally-transfused patients with thalassemia intermedia. *Haematologica* **2008**, *93*, 1095–1096. [CrossRef]
38. Olynyk, J.K.; St Pierre, T.G.; Britton, R.S.; Brunt, E.M.; Bacon, B.R. Duration of hepatic iron exposure increases the risk of significant fibrosis in hereditary hemochromatosis: A new role for magnetic resonance imaging. *Am. J. Gastroenterol.* **2005**, *100*, 837–841. [CrossRef]
39. Porter, J.B.; Cappellini, M.D.; Kattamis, A.; Viprakasit, V.; Mussalam, K.M.; Zhu, Z.; Taher, A.T. Iron overload across the spectrum of non-transfusion dependent thalassaemias: Role of erythropoiesis, splenectomy and transfusions. *Br. J. Haematol.* **2017**, *176*, 288–299. [CrossRef] [PubMed]
40. Taher, A.; Vichinsky, E.; Mussalam, K.M.; Cappellini, M.D.; Viprakasit, V. *Guidelines for the Management of Non-Transfusion Dependent Thalassaemia (NTDT)*, 2nd ed.; Thalassaemia International Federation: Nicosia, Cyprus, 2017.
41. Cappellini, M.D.; Cohen, A.; Porter, J.; Taher, A.; Viprakasit, V. *Guidelines for the Management of Transfusion Dependent Thalassaemia (TDT)*, 3rd ed.; Thalassaemia International Federation: Nicosia, Cyprus, 2014.
42. Piel, F. The present and future Global Burden of the inherited disorders of haemoglobin. *Hematol. Oncol. Clin. N. Am.* **2016**, *30*, 327–341. [CrossRef]
43. Kattamis, C.; Sofocleous, C.; Ladis, V.; Kattamis, A. Athens University thalassemia expertise unit: Evolution, structure, perspectives and patients' expectations. *Georgian Med. News* **2013**, *222*, 94–98.
44. Vives-Corrons, J.L.; Manu Pereira, M.M.; Romeo-Casabona, C.; Ncolas, P.; Gulbis, B.; Eleftheriou, A.; Angastiniotis, M.; Aguilar-Martinez, P.; Bianchi, P.; Van Wijk, R.; et al. Recommendations for centres of expertise in rare anaemias. The ENERCA White book. *Thalass. Rep.* **2014**, *4*, 4878.
45. EUCERD Recommendations for Centres of Expertise for Rare Diseases 2013. Available online: www.eucerd.eu (accessed on 20 March 2019).
46. Angastiniotis, M.; Eleftheriou, A.; Galanello, R.; Harteveld, C.L.; Petrou, M.; Traeger-Synodinos, J.; Giordano, P.; Jauniaux, E.; Modell, B.; Serour, G.; et al. *Prevention of Thalassaemias and Other Haemoglobin Disorders: Volume 1: Principles [Internet]*, 2nd ed.; Thalassaemia International Federation: Nicosia, Cyprus, 2013.
47. Cousens, N.E.; Gaff, C.L.; Metcalf, S.A.; Delatycki, M.B. Carrier screening for beta thalassaemia: A review of international practice. *Eur. J. Hum. Genet.* **2010**, *18*, 1077–1083. [CrossRef]

48. Koren, A.; Profeta, L.; Zalman, L.; Palmor, H.; Levin, C.; Zamir, R.B.; Shalev, S.; Blondheim, O. Prevention of β-thalassemia in Northern Israel—A Cost-Benefit Analysis. *Med. J. Hematol. Infect. Dis.* **2014**, *6*, e2014012. [CrossRef]
49. Allaf, B.; Patin, F.; Elion, J.; Couque, N. New approaches to accurate interpretation of sickle cell disease newborn screening by applying multiple of median cut offs and ratios. *Pediatr. Blood Cancer* **2018**, *65*, e27230. [CrossRef]
50. Rugless, M.J.; Fisher, C.A.; Stephens, A.D.; Amos, R.J.; Mohammed, T.; Old, J.M. Hb Bart's in cord blood: An accurate indicator of alpha-thalassemia. *Hemoglobin* **2006**, *30*, 57–62. [CrossRef]
51. Streely, A.; Latinovic, R.; Henthorn, J.; Daniel, Y.; Dormandy, E.; Darbyshire, P.; Mantio, D.; Fraser, L.; Farrar, L.; Will, A.; et al. Newborn blood spots results: Predictive value of screen positive test for thalassaemia major. *J. Med. Screen* **2013**, *20*, 183–187. [CrossRef]
52. Yu, C.; Huang, S.; Wang, M.; Zhang, J.; Liu, H.; Yuan, Z.; Wang, X.; He, X.; Wang, J.; Zou, L. A novel tandem mass spectrometry method for first line screening of mainly beta-thalassaemia from dried blood spots. *J. Proteom.* **2017**, *154*, 78–84. [CrossRef]

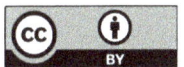

© 2019 by the authors. Licensee MDPI, Basel, Switzerland. This article is an open access article distributed under the terms and conditions of the Creative Commons Attribution (CC BY) license (http://creativecommons.org/licenses/by/4.0/).

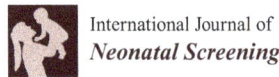

Review

Newborn Screening for Sickle Cell Disease and Other Hemoglobinopathies: A Short Review on Classical Laboratory Methods—Isoelectric Focusing, HPLC, and Capillary Electrophoresis

Claudia Frömmel [1,2]

1. MVZ Alexianer Labor GmbH, Große Hamburger Str. 5–11, 10115 Berlin, Germany; c.froemmel@alexianer.de; Tel.: +49-30-2311-2820
2. Newborn Screening Laboratory, Charité-Universitätsmedizin Berlin, Augustenburger Platz 1, 13353 Berlin, Germany

Received: 30 September 2018; Accepted: 1 November 2018; Published: 5 December 2018

Abstract: Sickle cell disease (SCD) and other hemoglobinopathies are a major health concern with a high burden of disease worldwide. Since the implementation of newborn screening (NBS) for SCD and other hemoglobinopathies in several regions of the world, technical progress of laboratory methods was achieved. This short review aims to summarize the current practice of classical laboratory methods for the detection of SCD and other hemoglobinopathies. This includes the newborn screening technologies of high-performance liquid chromatography (HPLC), capillary electrophoresis (CE), and isoelectric focusing (IEF).

Keywords: newborn screening; sickle cell disease; hemoglobinopathy; laboratory methods; neonatal screening; hemoglobin pattern; HPLC; IEF; capillary electrophoresis

1. Introduction

Newborn screening (NBS) for sickle cell disease (SCD) as one element of prevention programs for hemoglobinopathies has been in place in several regions in the world for more than 40 years now. First attempts were made in the United States of America (USA) and Jamaica, as well as in Great Britain in the 1970s [1,2]. Starting with alkaline electrophoresis, the development of faster and more precise methods permitted the development of extended and more sophisticated prevention programs of hemoglobinopathies. The aim of NBS for SCD is to prevent major health complications of SCD from early childhood onward. SCD in this context comprises all forms of relevant sickling disorders, originating from different genetic constellations (e.g., homozygous HbS (HbSS) and compound heterozygous forms as HbS/β^0 thalassemia, HbS/β^+ thalassemia, HbS/HbC, HbS/HbD^{Punjab}, HbS/HbE, HbS/HbO^{Arab}, HbS/Hb Lepore, and HbS/$\delta\beta$ thalassemia). As life-threatening events can occur in children with SCD from three months of age onward, early diagnosis is desirable to establish preventive measures. Patients with thalassemia and other major hemoglobin disorders do not benefit in the same way from early diagnosis. However, these disorders have important implications for family health, and the burden of disease is very high in several regions of the world, thus demanding preventive action. In this context, many newborn screening programs make use of the possibility to detect carriers of hemoglobin variants as a by-product to provide families with reproductive knowledge and informed decision-making regarding hemoglobinopathies.

Laboratory methods to detect disease states and carrier states (if included in the program) should be very sensitive and highly specific. To prevent harm, they should not miss patients and should not falsely identify patients. Psychosocial and logistic burdens to families from screening or diagnostic evaluation, an increased risk of unnecessary medical treatment, or a delayed diagnosis from false negative results, as well as psychosocial harm from false positive results and uncertainty of clinical diagnosis, should be minimized and be outweighed by the benefits [3].

While laboratories for newborn screening for endocrine and metabolic disorders mainly use tandem mass spectrometry (MS/MS) or photometric assays, technologies, which are commonly established for NBS for hemoglobinopathies include HPLC, isoelectric focusing (IEF), and capillary electrophoresis (CE). They were developed for larger sample sizes from routine hemoglobinopathy testing and permit the clear separation of hemoglobin variants of interest in an automated or semi-automated way. Recent developments of screening methods like tandem mass spectrometry (MS/MS) and Matrix-assisted laser desorption/ionization time-of-flight mass spectrometry (MALDI-TOF MS) or molecular genetic testing are explained elsewhere.

2. Technologies

Technologies are based on the separation of hemoglobin species (Hb) and the quantification of respective hemoglobin fractions from dried blood spot (DBS) or fresh cord blood samples. They should be able to detect HbS and HbC, and separate HbF and HbA, as well as being able to detect other hemoglobin variants of clinical relevance, such as HbD^{Punjab}, HbE, Hb Lepore, and HbO^{Arab}. The screening methods reviewed here provide provisional results and identify putative abnormal fractions of hemoglobin and have to be confirmed to give a definite diagnosis.

In contrast to the diagnosis of carriers and patients with hemoglobinopathies in clinical routine or carrier screening programs, where a complete blood count with erythrocyte indices and parameters of iron metabolism are included, newborn screening is only based on the separation of hemoglobin from DBS or cord blood. Additional tests such as the solubility test for HbS are not applicable. As symptoms usually do not occur before two months of age, results of screening should be provided within this period. An algorithm designed to clearly state when parents should be informed and a defined follow-up help avoid reduced effectiveness of the whole process.

2.1. HPLC

Automated cation-exchange high-performance liquid chromatography (HPLC) is a widely used method to screen for hemoglobinopathies with a clear separation and quantification of hemoglobin fractions [4–11]. The method is based on the elution of hemoglobin bound to a solid phase over time by buffers with a pH gradient. The time from the injection of the sample into the column to the elution of the hemoglobin fraction is called the retention time. Eluted hemoglobin is detected by a dual-wavelength detector and quantified by integrating the area under curve of the produced chromatogram, expressed as a percentage of the total area (Figure 1). A characteristic retention time (window of detection), together with the relative quantification, permits presumptive identification of all relevant hemoglobin species: HbF, HbA, HbA$_2$, HbS, HbC, HbD^{Punjab}, HbE, Hb Lepore, and HbO^{Arab}. Hb Bart's is also detected. HPLC analysis is very precise and reproducible with an inter-run coefficient of variation (CV) of <5%. The detection limit for HbA and HbS was shown to be around 1% of total hemoglobin [4,6,12]. Calibrators and material for internal quality assurance containing Hb FAES and FADC (where letters represent different Hb species) are available.

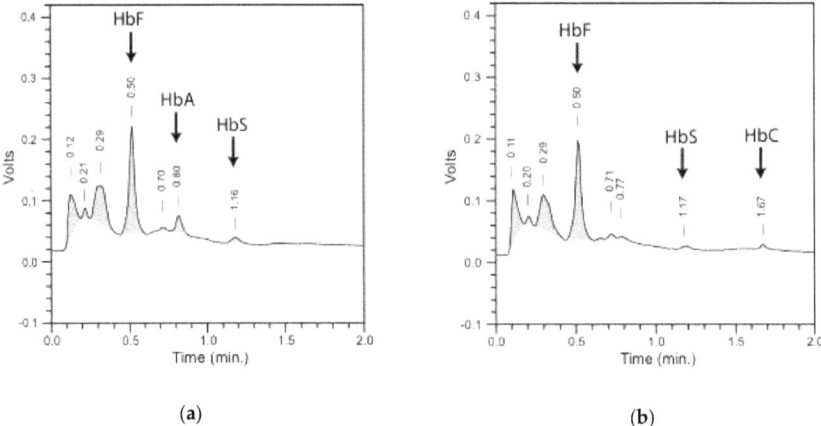

Figure 1. Chromatogram of HPLC (Variant™ newborn screening (nbs), Bio-Rad laboratories, Europe): the x-axis represents the time in minutes, and the y-axis represents the response in volts; retention times of integrated peaks are shown above the peaks, and peaks of Hb variants included in the pattern are named and indicated with an arrow: (**a**) pattern of HbF/HbA/HbS (FAS); (**b**) pattern of HbF/HbS/HbC (FSC).

2.2. CE

Capillary electrophoresis (CE) combines two principles of separation of hemoglobins, the electrophoretic mobility in alkaline buffer and the electro-osmotic flow resulting in excellent separation. High voltage applied to an in silica glass capillary prompt hemoglobin molecules to migrate toward a detector of 415-nm wavelength. Detected hemoglobin fractions can be relatively quantified and produce a pherogram. HbF is centered in the neonatal system (note: it is HbA in the adult system), followed by the automated integration of peaks and defined migration zones (N1 to N13—specific to the neonatal system) which allow the easy interpretation of pherograms and help identify hemoglobin patterns (Figure 2).

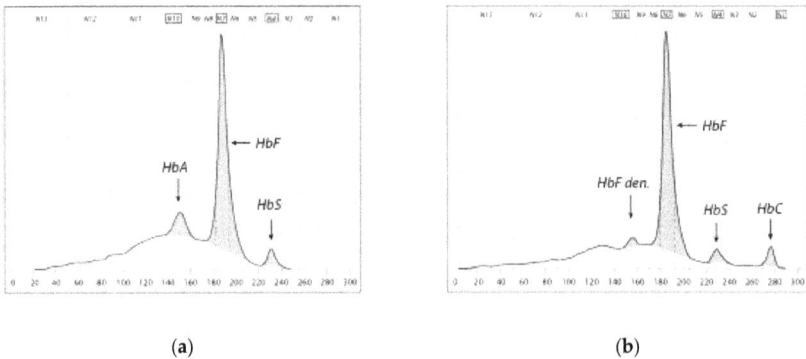

Figure 2. Pherogram of capillary electrophoresis (CE; Capillarys™ neonat fast, Sebia, France); zone from left to right: N13–N1. Peaks of Hb variants included in the pattern are named: (**a**) pattern of FAS; (**b**) pattern of FSC.

CE is able to detect and relatively quantify HbF, HbA, HbA$_2$, HbS, HbC, HbD^{Punjab}, HbO^{Arab}, HbE, and Hb Lepore. Hb Bart's is also detected. Many other Hb variants may be detected including γ- and α-chain abnormalities with an overlap in the zones of the more common hemoglobins, e.g.,

HbD^{Punjab} and Hb Korle Bu in zone N5 [13]. Interpretation has to be diligent with regards to reporting named hemoglobin variants following the presumptive identification of the system. Controls for internal quality assurance are provided containing HbF, HbA, HbS and HbC. The detection limit for HbA and HbS was found to be around 1% of total hemoglobin.

2.3. IEF

IEF is a very sensitive method and is widely used at relatively low costs. IEF separates hemoglobin species according to their isoelectric point on a gel medium with very high resolution. Hb variants migrate in a pH gradient to the point where their net charge becomes zero. Bands are narrow compared to classical electrophoresis and give a precise picture (Figure 3). HbF and HbA, as well as relevant hemoglobins HbS, HbC, HbD^{Punjab}, HbE, and HbO^{Arab}, can be separated. Hb Bart's can also be detected. IEF separates post-translationally modified variants, which sometimes makes interpretation difficult; thus, an experienced staff is needed to read results.

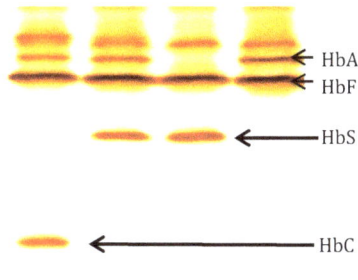

Figure 3. Isoelectric focusing gel picture (RESOLVE™, Perkin Elmer, Finland); from left to right: patterns of FAC, FAS, FS, and FA, adopted from Reference [14].

IEF is a semi-automated system, which allows the parallel run of several gels entailing some labor-intensive steps. Easier work-up and documentation of gels are achieved using a scanning software. Controls for internal quality assurance contain HbF, HbA, HbS and HbC.

3. Interpretation of Newborn Screening Results and Hemoglobin Patterns

Normal newborn samples mainly contain HbF ($\alpha 2/\gamma 2$) and a smaller amount of HbA ($\alpha 2/\beta 2$). HbA levels range from 6 to 40% with an average of 19%, showing inter-individual variations. HbA levels in newborns are dependent on gestational age and date of sampling, reflecting the stage of hemoglobin switch [6,12]. In Table 1, patterns of the detected hemoglobins are listed in the order of highest percentage to the lowest. One has to be aware that relevant Hb variants may present an abnormal pattern similar to those consistent with a target disease. Today, there are more than 1000 variants of hemoglobin known. Software solutions for HPLC and CE suggest a pattern, which has to be verified by the technician reviewing the chromatogram or pherogram. In IEF, an experienced staff reviews the gel, and densitometry helps quantify hemoglobin variants to determine the pattern. Guidelines and lab handbooks can be used to interpret hemoglobin patterns, specifying the significance of a found pattern and the possible pitfalls according to the methods applied. An abnormal result with the screening method (first line) is repeated from the sample using a secondary method (second line), or using the same method if another is not available.

Table 1. Hemoglobinopathies relevant in newborn screening (NBS) and their respective patterns.

Target Disease	Pattern	
Sickle cell disease Primary target		
HbSS,	FS [1]	
HbS/β^0 thalassemia,		
HbS/$\delta\beta$ thalassemia,		
HbS/HPFH		
HbS/C	FSC	
HbS/β^+ thalassemia	FSA	
HbS/D^{Punjab}	FSD [2]	
HbS/E	FSE	
HbS/other variant [3]	FSX	
Thalassemia syndromes and other hemoglobinopathies		Secondary target
β^0 thalassemia	F only	
β^+ thalassemia	FA [4]	
HbEE	FE	
HbE/β^0 thalassemia		
HbE/β^+ thalassemia	FEA	
HbCC or	FC	
HbC/β^0 thalassemia		
HbC/β^+ thalassemia	FCA	
HbDD^{Punjab} or	FD	
HbD^{Punjab}/β^0 thalassemia		
HbD^{Punjab}/β^+ thalassemia	FDA	
Hb variant not specified homozygous	FX	
Hb variant/β^0 or β^+ thalassemia	FXA	
Severe α thalassemia,	FABart's [5]	
HbH disease		
Severe α thalassemia,	FE Bart's (e.g)	
HbH disease with other variants [6]	FAX Bart's	
Traits Secondary target		
HbS	FAS	
HbD^{Punjab}	FAD	
HbC	FAC	
HbE	FAE	
Other Hb variant [7]	FAX	
Normal	FA	

[1] Hb variants migrating similarly to HbS may be hidden; [2] HbD has to be verified as HbD^{Punjab}, as many other variants run like HbD^{Punjab}; [3] Hb variants not specified during screening, or specified with second-line methods, e.g., Hb Lepore, or HbO^{Arab} if included in the program; [4] HbA <5% or <1.5% (overlap of premature newborns and normal newborns) depend on cut-off used; [5] detected Hb Bart's (over cut-off or qualitative); [6] includes detected Hb Bart's with combined α- or β-variants and, e.g., HbE with Hb Bart's; [7] Hb variants not specified during screening or specified with second-line methods, e.g., Hb Lepore, or HbO^{Arab} if included in the program.

3.1. Target Diseases

Patients with sickle cell disease and non-sickling disorders, as well as carriers of abnormal hemoglobin variants, can be detected by NBS. Choosing primary and secondary target diseases influences false negative and false positive results of the overall screening program and, therefore, are important to the evaluation of the screening process. NBS for hemoglobinopathies has sensitivity and specificity close to 100% for SCD with regards to the different genetic forms defined as target diseases (see below); however, it loses sensitivity and specificity when non-sickling disorders are included. Furthermore, pre-analytic factors like prematurity and blood transfusions prior to sampling influence the sensitivity. The positive and negative predictive values vary with prevalence of the abnormal variants and thalassemia syndromes.

3.2. Sickle Cell Disease

Sickle cell disease is a severe hematological disorder with acute and chronic manifestations caused by a complex pathomechanism of hemolysis and recurrent vaso-occlusive events. Life-threatening early complications can be largely avoided by initiating simple and effective prophylactic measures such as penicillin, vaccination, and parent education. Primary target diseases are all common and are generally severe sickling disorders (see Table 1).

HbS/hereditary persistence of fetal hemoglobin (HPFH) is included as a very mild disorder, as it cannot be distinguished from homozygous HbS and β^0 thalassemia/HbS. This is accepted, as the disorder seems relatively rare. The definite diagnosis should be ruled out by confirmatory diagnostics for appropriate counseling and treatment [15].

For the distinction between the disease states of HbS/β^+ thalassemia or HbS/β^{++} thalassemia and a simple carrier state for HbS, the relative quantification of HbA and HbS and the ratio between HbA/HbS is used (mainly a cut-off of <1). This approach bears the risk of false positive and false negative results, as there is an overlap between HbS/β^+ thalassemia or HbS/β^{++} thalassemia and a simple carrier state for HbS, especially in premature babies. In these cases, HbA is present, but at different levels depending on gestational age. Additionally, precise quantification is a problem close to the detection limit of a variant for HPLC and CE [5,7]. To standardize quantitative interpretation of screening results, cut-offs and ratios can be expressed as multiples of median (MoM) [12]. IEF is a method with a very high resolution, but it sometimes hampers precise quantification and correct classification of bands, and there is a slight tendency to over-detect variants of no significance, e.g., modified HbA or γ-variants [5,16].

For all described methods, there are difficulties due to the fact that, with over 1000 known abnormal Hb variants, some of them will migrate, differently from HbA, but together with HbS or other common variants (HbC, HbD, and HbE). Genetic constellations like Hb Hope and HbS can lead to false positive screening results for SCD, which can then be excluded by a second-line method or by confirmatory testing [17]. Unusual analytical pictures may occur, depending on whether these rare abnormal variants with migration properties similar to HbS (or other common variants) derive from γ-, α-, or β-globin chain mutations. Heterozygous α-globin chain variants produce additional peaks or bands and comprise about one-fourth of HbF and HbA (or HbS if an additional β-mutation is present) if all four α-genes are functional, or about one-third if one α-gene is missing, or one-half if two α-genes are missing, provided the α-variant is stable. From all possible genotypes for SCD, the suitable target diseases should be defined according to the whole screening process, in both the screening laboratory and the confirmatory laboratory. With regards to this definition, cases of SCD caused by very rare genotypes, such as dominant HbS with a double mutation, are missed by classical NBS [17]; moreover, milder disorders such as HbS/β^{++} thalassemia or HbS/HPFH might be detected.

3.3. Non-Sickling Disorders

Other hemoglobinopathies with clinical relevance, including severe disorders such as β-thalassemia major and severe α-thalassemia (HbH disease), are often also included in NBS for SCD as secondary target diseases.

3.3.1. β-Thalassemia Major and Intermedia

β-thalassemia major or intermedia results from homozygous or compound heterozygous β^0 or β^+ mutations. Patients suffer from severe anemia, which requires regular or irregular blood transfusion and chelation therapy to prevent iron overload. Early detection is wanted to prevent babies from becoming severely anemic and to support family health in social and medical aspects by giving the possibility of informed choice for future pregnancies and by including the affected child in a comprehensive care program for thalassemia. β-thalassemia major can be expected in samples with a hemoglobin pattern of HbF only, or HbF and HbA below a certain cut-off from 0–5% (<1.5% in the United Kingdom (UK)) [18,19].

3.3.2. Severe α-Thalassemia, HbH Disease

HbH disease has a variable phenotype ranging from mild microcytic anemia to severe transfusion-dependent anemia. HbH disease is caused by deletion or inactivation of three α-globin genes with an imbalance of chain synthesis, leading to the association of β-chains in adults (β2/β2), known as HbH, and of γ-chains in newborns, known as Hb Bart's (γ2/γ2). Clinically significant hemolytic anemia, which possibly necessitates blood transfusion, can occur during fever, infections, and pregnancy. Severe aplastic crises after infection with parvovirus B19 or growth retardation during childhood, as well as iron overload in adults with or without previous transfusion, are possible complications in a minority of patients. In regions with high prevalence and also in some low prevalence areas for α-thalassemia, HbH disease is included in the newborn screening program as a target disease. Technologies such as IEF, HPLC, and CE are able to detect Hb Bart's [20–24]. Several cut-offs were evaluated for HPLC or a qualitative detection of Hb Bart's in the fraction of fast-eluting hemoglobins ($\geq$15% or $\geq$20% or $\geq$25% for the FAST fraction on the Bio-Rad™ nbs System, evaluated on different integration principles). IEF and CE represent a qualitative analysis of Hb Bart's. Detection of Hb Bart's shows considerable overlap between HbH disease and heterozygous α^0 thalassemia. Literature about the sensitivity and the specificity for Hb Bart's is scarce. Specificity seems lower than that for β-thalassemia and positive predictive values in a low-prevalence region will be unsatisfactory. Screening policy should decide on whether false negative results outweigh false positive results or vice versa. As Hb Bart's is unstable, sensitivity also depends on material (DBS vs. fresh-cord blood), the day of sampling, and the storage of samples until measurement.

Including HbH disease in a neonatal screening setting is still controversial, as over-diagnosis is probable [20]. It seems more acceptable in high-prevalence areas and if the definite diagnosis by verifying deletional and/or non-deletional α-thalassemia through DNA analysis is done in the screening center [10,23]. Asian publications show a higher detection rate using DNA analysis in the first line [25].

3.4. Carrier Detection

With IEF, CE, and HPLC, carriers of relevant Hb variants can be incidentally detected. HPLC and CE provide presumptive identification of a variant. Variant peaks occur in their respective windows or zones and, together with the percentages of HbA and the variant peak, a presumptive result can be reported. All screening programs which include carrier detection recommend two independent methods as first- and second-line laboratory methods (e.g., IEF and HPLC or HPLC and CE). Whereas carriers of heterozygous β-thalassemia are not detectable in newborns by measurement of HbA_2, the measurement of HbA and a cut-off <15% may be indicative for the β-thalassemia trait in newborns [19]. Confirmatory diagnostic follow-ups using a new sample with blood count, hemoglobin separation analysis, and, if necessary, DNA analysis then provide a definite result. These inexpensive methods can be used for carrier detection to improve family health, as well as in states where no antenatal screening program is in place; however, they can also lead to stigmatization and counterproductive effects [26–28].

4. Pre-Analytics

Limitations of the aforementioned methods lie often in the pre-analytical phase. The used material can be fresh cord blood or dried blood spot from a heel prick. Storage of cord blood should not exceed seven days at 4 °C and that of dried blood spots should not exceed 1 month. Older samples show lower elution of samples from the DBS and, often, the degradation of hemoglobin, resulting in a high baseline, increased noise, and unclear peaks with difficulties in zone adjustment and quantification, especially in Hb species present at low percentage.

Blood from premature babies contains lower percentages of HbA or other β-chain variants, which may lead to false negative results in screening for SCD. Although an exact gestational age for requesting a second sample is not defined, premature babies under 33 weeks of gestational age should receive repeated testing.

Babies who received blood transfusions show increased percentages of adult hemoglobin HbA and HbA_2 and the presence of a severe hemoglobinopathy may be masked. Therefore, it seems essential that transfused babies can be identified using either HbA levels above the 2.5 multiples of median (MoM) dependent on gestational age or ratios of HbF/HbA [12].

5. Conclusions

HPLC, CE, and IEF have proven to be suitable methods for NBS for sickle cell disease and other hemoglobinopathies in several different states and regions with specific legal and economic conditions. They have very high sensitivity and high specificity regarding SCD with patterns of FS, FSC, and FSE, and just slightly lower for patterns of FSA and FSD. Other non-sickling hemoglobinopathies were successfully included in newborn screening programs, and future developments must match the achievements of this recent era of hemoglobin analysis systems and will add new flexibility.

Funding: This research did not receive any specific funding in the public, commercial, or non-profit sectors.

Acknowledgments: I would like to thank Stephan Lobitz and Jeanette Klein for their constant support, Cornelius Frömmel, Bryony Fox, and Daniel Wiesenfeld for their help with the manuscript, Barbara Wild for providing the gel picture and Thomas Burmeister for assistance refining the figures. Cornelis Harteveld and Bichr Allaf for helpful discussions, and Annemarie Brose for technical advice.

Conflicts of Interest: The author declares no conflicts of interest.

References

1. Serjeant, B.E.; Forbes, M.; Williams, L.L.; Serjeant, G.R. Screening cord bloods for detection of sickle cell disease in Jamaica. *Clin. Chem.* **1974**, *20*, 666–669. [PubMed]
2. Pearson, H.A.; O'Brien, R.T.; McLntosh, S.; Aspnes, G.T.; Yang, M. Routine screening of umbilical cord blood for sickle cell diseases. *JAMA* **1974**, *227*, 420–421. [CrossRef] [PubMed]
3. Goldenberg, A.J.; Comeau, A.M.; Grosse, S.D.; Tanksley, S.; Prosser, L.A.; Ojodu, J.; Botkin, J.R.; Kemper, A.R.; Green, N.S. Evaluating Harms in the Assessment of Net Benefit: A Framework for Newborn Screening Condition Review. *Matern. Child Health J.* **2016**, *20*, 693–700. [CrossRef] [PubMed]
4. Eastman, J.W.; Wong, R.; Liao, C.L.; Morales, D.R. Automated HPLC screening of newborns for sickle cell anemia and other hemoglobinopathies. *Clin. Chem.* **1996**, *42*, 704–710. [CrossRef]
5. Campbell, M.; Henthorn, J.S.; Davies, S.C. Evaluation of cation-exchange HPLC compared with isoelectric focusing for neonatal hemoglobinopathy screening. *Clin. Chem.* **1999**, *45*, 969–975.
6. Bouva, M.J.; Mohrmann, K.; Brinkman, H.B.; Kemper-Proper, E.A.; Elvers, B.; Loeber, J.G.; Verheul, F.E.; Giordano, P.C. Implementing neonatal screening for haemoglobinopathies in the Netherlands. *J. Med. Screen.* **2010**, *17*, 58–65. [CrossRef] [PubMed]
7. Frommel, C.; Brose, A.; Klein, J.; Blankenstein, O.; Lobitz, S. Newborn screening for sickle cell disease: Technical and legal aspects of a German pilot study with 38,220 participants. *BioMed Res. Int.* **2014**, *2014*, 695828–695838. [CrossRef] [PubMed]
8. Greene, D.N.; Pyle, A.L.; Chang, J.S.; Hoke, C.; Lorey, T. Comparison of Sebia Capillarys Flex capillary electrophoresis with the BioRad Variant II high pressure liquid chromatography in the evaluation of hemoglobinopathies. *Clin. Chim. Acta* **2012**, *413*, 1232–1238. [CrossRef] [PubMed]
9. Lorey, F.; Cunningham, G.; Shafer, F.; Lubin, B.; Vichinsky, E. Universal screening for hemoglobinopathies using high-performance liquid chromatography: Clinical results of 2.2 million screens. *Eur. J. Hum. Genet.* **1994**, *2*, 262–271. [CrossRef] [PubMed]

10. Hoppe, C.C. Newborn screening for hemoglobin disorders. *Hemoglobin* **2011**, *35*, 556–564. [CrossRef] [PubMed]
11. Upadhye, D.S.; Jain, D.L.; Trivedi, Y.L.; Nadkarni, A.H.; Ghosh, K.; Colah, R.B. Newborn screening for haemoglobinopathies by high performance liquid chromatography (HPLC): Diagnostic utility of different approaches in resource-poor settings. *Clin. Chem. Lab. Med.* **2014**, *52*, 1791–1796. [CrossRef] [PubMed]
12. Allaf, B.; Patin, F.; Elion, J.; Couque, N. New approach to accurate interpretation of sickle cell disease newborn screening by applying multiple of median cutoffs and ratios. *Pediatr. Blood Cancer* **2018**, *65*, e27230. [CrossRef] [PubMed]
13. Renom, G.; Mereau, C.; Maboudou, P.; Perini, J.M. Potential of the Sebia Capillarys neonat fast automated system for neonatal screening of sickle cell disease. *Clin. Chem. Lab. Med.* **2009**, *47*, 1423–1432. [CrossRef] [PubMed]
14. Wild, B. The Haemoglobinopathies: Learning from EQA, UK NEQAS. Available online: https://www.ukneqash.org/documents.php (accessed on 29 September 2018).
15. Serjeant, G.R.; Serjeant, B.E.; Hambleton, I.R.; Oakley, M.; Thein, S.L.; Clark, B. A Plea for the Newborn Diagnosis of Hb S-Hereditary Persistence of Fetal Hemoglobin. *Hemoglobin* **2017**, *41*, 216–217. [CrossRef] [PubMed]
16. Hustace, T.; Fleisher, J.M.; Sanchez Varela, A.M.; Podda, A.; Alvarez, O. Increased prevalence of false positive hemoglobinopathy newborn screening in premature infants. *Pediatr. Blood Cancer* **2011**, *57*, 1039–1043. [CrossRef] [PubMed]
17. Moradkhani, K.; Riou, J.; Wajcman, H. Pitfalls in the genetic diagnosis of Hb S. *Clin. Biochem.* **2013**, *46*, 291–299. [CrossRef] [PubMed]
18. Ryan, K.; Bain, B.J.; Worthington, D.; James, J.; Plews, D.; Mason, A.; Roper, D.; Rees, D.C.; de la Salle, B.; Streetly, A. Significant haemoglobinopathies: Guidelines for screening and diagnosis. *Br. J. Haematol.* **2010**, *149*, 35–49. [CrossRef]
19. Mantikou, E.; Arkesteijn, S.G.; Beckhoven van, J.M.; Kerkhoffs, J.L.; Harteveld, C.L.; Giordano, P.C. A brief review on newborn screening methods for hemoglobinopathies and preliminary results selecting beta thalassemia carriers at birth by quantitative estimation of the HbA fraction. *Clin. Biochem.* **2009**, *42*, 1780–1785. [CrossRef] [PubMed]
20. Bouva, M.J.; Sollaino, C.; Perseu, L.; Galanello, R.; Giordano, P.C.; Harteveld, C.L.; Cnossen, M.H.; Schielen, P.C.; Elvers, L.H.; Peters, M. Relationship between neonatal screening results by HPLC and the number of alpha-thalassaemia gene mutations; consequences for the cut-off value. *J. Med. Screen.* **2011**, *18*, 182–186. [CrossRef] [PubMed]
21. Jindatanmanusan, P.; Riolueang, S.; Glomglao, W.; Sukontharangsri, Y.; Chamnanvanakij, S.; Torcharus, K.; Viprakasit, V. Diagnostic applications of newborn screening for alpha-thalassaemias, haemoglobins E and H disorders using isoelectric focusing on dry blood spots. *Ann. Clin. Biochem.* **2014**, *51*, 237–247. [CrossRef]
22. Liao, C.; Zhou, J.Y.; Xie, X.M.; Tang, H.S.; Li, R.; Li, D.Z. Newborn screening for Hb H disease by determination of Hb Bart's using the Sebia capillary electrophoresis system in southern China. *Hemoglobin* **2014**, *38*, 73–75. [CrossRef] [PubMed]
23. Uaprasert, N.; Settapiboon, R.; Amornsiriwat, S.; Sarnthammakul, P.; Thanapat, T.; Rojnuckarin, P.; Sutcharitchan, P. Diagnostic utility of isoelectric focusing and high performance liquid chromatography in neonatal cord blood screening for thalassemia and non-sickling hemoglobinopathies. *Clin. Chim. Acta* **2014**, *427*, 23–26. [CrossRef] [PubMed]
24. Rugless, M.J.; Fisher, C.A.; Stephens, A.D.; Amos, R.J.; Mohammed, T.; Old, J.M. Hb Bart's in cord blood: An accurate indicator of alpha-thalassemia. *Hemoglobin* **2006**, *30*, 57–62. [CrossRef]
25. Wu, M.Y.; Xie, X.M.; Li, J., Li, D.Z. Neonatal screening for alpha-thalassemia by cord hemoglobin Barts: How effective is it? *Int. J. Lab. Hematol.* **2015**, *37*, 649–653. [CrossRef] [PubMed]
26. Bain, B.J. Haemoglobinopathy diagnosis: Algorithms, lessons and pitfalls. *Blood Rev.* **2011**, *25*, 205–213. [CrossRef] [PubMed]

27. Bombard, Y.; Miller, F.A.; Hayeems, R.Z.; Wilson, B.J.; Carroll, J.C.; Paynter, M.; Little, J.; Allanson, J.; Bytautas, J.P.; Chakraborty, P. Health-care providers' views on pursuing reproductive benefit through newborn screening: The case of sickle cell disorders. *Eur. J. Hum. Genet.* **2012**, *20*, 498–504. [CrossRef] [PubMed]
28. Ross, L.F. Newborn screening for sickle cell disease: Whose reproductive benefit? *Eur. J. Hum. Genet.* **2012**, *20*, 484–485. [CrossRef]

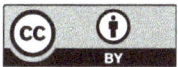

© 2018 by the author. Licensee MDPI, Basel, Switzerland. This article is an open access article distributed under the terms and conditions of the Creative Commons Attribution (CC BY) license (http://creativecommons.org/licenses/by/4.0/).

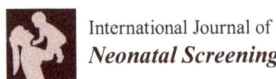

Review

Newborn Sickle Cell Disease Screening Using Electrospray Tandem Mass Spectrometry

Yvonne Daniel [1],* and Charles Turner [2]

1. Viapath, Guy's & St Thomas Hospital, London SE17EH, UK
2. WellChild Laboratory, Evelina London Children's Hospital, London SE17EH, UK; Charles.turner@gstt.nhs.uk
* Correspondence: yvonne.daniel@viapath.co.uk

Received: 7 September 2018; Accepted: 22 November 2018; Published: 24 November 2018

Abstract: There is a growing demand for newborn sickle cell disease screening globally. Historically techniques have relied on the separation of intact haemoglobin tetramers using electrophoretic or liquid chromatography techniques. These techniques also identify haemoglobin variants of no clinical significance. Specific electrospray ionization-mass spectrometry-mass spectrometry techniques to analyse targeted peptides formed after digestion of the haemoglobin with trypsin were reported in 2005. Since this time the method has been further developed and adopted in several European countries. It is estimated that more than one million babies have been screened with no false-negative cases reported. This review reports on the current use of the technique and reviews the related publications.

Keywords: screening; sickle cell disease; newborn; mass spectrometry

1. Introduction

The first report of newborn screening for sickle cell disease (SCD) by mass spectrometry (MS) utilised matrix-assisted laser desorption-time of flight (MALDI-TOF) [1]. Intact haemoglobin chains were initially analysed followed by mass mapping of trypsin-active MS targets to localise the mutation site. This proof of concept had not translated into large-scale trials or prospective screening until recently. Newborn screening using MALDI-TOF is covered in a separate article in this issue and it will not be reviewed further here. The other ionisation mode for MS in common use is electrospray ionisation (ESI). ESI of undigested haemoglobin produces a large number of multiply charged ions, formed in the source when charged droplets are dried in the presence of an inert gas such as nitrogen. The ions formed can then be analysed.

Wild et al. [2] reported the use of ESI-MS to analyse intact globin chains in 147 newborn blood spots. The protocol utilised software to produce a deconvoluted profile spectrum displaying the α, β, and γ globin peaks along with peaks of variant haemoglobins with a mass shift sufficiently different from normal to allow resolution. This allowed detection of sickle globin and other variants with a mass difference of −30 daltons (Da) from normal β chains but did not clearly resolve those clinically significant variants with a mass difference of 1 Da. The method was not specific for Hb S, as there are 5 amino acid substitutions which result in a mass difference of 30 Da. The authors concluded that the technique allowed for detection of sickle cell disease, but samples found to have a positive signal for Hb S would require confirmation by an alternate technique. No large-scale trial of this ESI-MS approach has been published. In 2005, Daniel et al. [3] published the first report of a targeted ESI-MSMS approach, based on tryptic digestion. Developments of this method have been widely adopted into active newborn screening programmes and are the main subject of this review.

2. The MSMS (Tandem Mass Spectrometry) Technique

ESI coupled to tandem mass spectrometry (MSMS), in which ions formed are selected in a first quadrupole (Q1), product ions are produced via collision in Q2 and detected in Q3, is in common use in newborn screening for small molecules such as amino acids and acylcarnitiines. The 2005 paper of Daniel et al. [3] achieved targeted detection of haemoglobin variants including clinically significant variants with 1 Da mass difference from normal using ESI-MSMS with a series of experiments run simultaneously on whole blood samples digested with trypsin. Trypsin cleaves peptide bonds adjacent to arginine and lysine residues producing a predictable and reproducible series of peptide fragments. As the clinically significant haemoglobin variants have been well characterised, the amino acid sequences are known along with the expected mass differences from normal. The target beta chain haemoglobin variants were Hb S and Hb C, Hb D^{Punjab} and Hb O^{Arab}, and Hb E which occur in tryptic peptides (T) 1, 13, and 3 respectively. Selected reaction monitoring experiments were designed to select the required tryptic peptide in Q1 and a specific fragmentation ion in Q3 generated following collision induced fragmentation in Q2. Experiments were designed for wildtype and the designated haemoglobin variants. Unlike the previous method using intact chains, this method was targeted and highly specific. Additionally, the use of ESI-MSMS allowed rationalisation of equipment and better use of existing resources. The tryptic digestion had been simplified by the demonstration that informative peptides were produced within 30–45 min and that chemical denaturation of the protein or purification of haemoglobin prior to the addition of trypsin was unnecessary. A patent was awarded to the final method in 2006. The method of Daniel et al. [3] was commercialised by SpOtOn Clinical Diagnostics from 2013, and CE-marked reagent kits were made available in 2015. The kits include stable isotope-labeled Hb S peptide and trypsin, and peptide standards for instrument optimization are also available from the company. Dried blood spot samples are punched (3 mm spot), stable isotope and trypsin are added, and the samples incubated at 37 °C for 30 min. Following the addition of mobile phase to stop the reaction and act as diluent, samples are introduced into the MSMS using flow injection (without chromatography). The method utilizes simple acetonitrile/water/formic acid mobile phases as used for newborn screening for amino acids and acyl carnitines. The stable isotope-labeled Hb S allows sample-by-sample assurance of trypsin activity and MSMS performance.

3. Review of Published Results

The initial method was validated in a project funded by the NHS Sickle Cell & Thalassaemia Screening programme, which compared newborn blood spots analysed by the existing isoelectric focussing technique (IEF) in Leeds with the ESI-MSMS technique [4]. Over 40,000 blood spots were tested between August 2007 and August 2008. The results were analysed by reviewing the abundance ratio of the variant peptide to the corresponding wild-type peptide with no discrepant results observed, shown in Table 1.

Subsequently Boemer et al. [5] reported the results of 2082 newborn samples screened using a slightly modified MSMS method with the same principle. Results were compared with IEF and high performance liquid chromatography (HPLC). Only haemoglobins S, C, E, and wild-type β and γ were targeted with multiple experiments for each haemoglobin of interest. No discrepancies were reported. In 2011, the group reported a review of three years' experience presenting the results of 43,736 newborn samples [6]. First-line MSMS analysis identified 444 samples as screen-positive. All were confirmed using molecular techniques. The paper also reported ranges obtained for the amalgamated ratio data of the variant to corresponding wild-type peptides as well as the β to γ peptides used to screen for β thalassaemia disease. These showed clear discrimination between unaffected and affected cases within each of the investigated disease categories, as well as carriers for the haemoglobin variants. The group noted the lack of an experiment to detect Hb Bart's and therefore possible Hb H disease and noted the possibility that Hb S co-inherited with other clinically significant variants not targeted in the experimental protocol would have a result pattern identical to that of a sickle carrier.

Table 1. Results of comparison of blood spots and the isoelectric focussing technique (IEF).

Haemoglobins Detected	Number (n)
Total samples tested	40,054
No abnormality detected	39,710
FS	9
FSC	3
FC	1
FAS	187
FAC	38
FAD^{Punjab}	49
FAE	47
FAO^{Arab}	0
Wild-type β absent [#]	4

F = fetal; A = adult/wild type; [#] all subsequently confirmed as β thalassaemia disease.

Moat et al. [7] used the SpOtOn kit method in a study to inform the introduction of newborn screening for sickle cell disease in Wales. The published protocol built on the use of ratios and utilised locked software algorithms to screen for sickle cell and β thalassaemia disease, the latter as a clinically significant by-product. The only parameters available and routinely reviewed by the operator were those required to check for appropriate tryptic sample digestion, prematurity, and transfusion status. The developed algorithms prevented the identification of most sickle cell carriers and all carriers and homozygotes of C, D^{Punjab}, O^{Arab}, and E, as the operator was not alerted to the results of these experiments unless Hb S was detected at levels above the designated ratio action values. Ratio action values were set using the residual blood spots of 2154 normal and 675 known positive cases and were subsequently evaluated using 13,249 blood spots run in parallel with HPLC. The protocol identified some Hb S carriers as ratio action values were set sufficiently low to ensure that all possible cases of coinheritance of Hb S and β plus thalassaemia were detected. Unblinding of the data revealed a further 328 cases of infants who were carriers of either Hb S, C, D^{Punjab}, or E, which had not been identified to the operator using the locked protocol. As the protocol is designed not to identify cases that are carriers of Hb S, it does not permit the detection of rare Hb variants that interact with Hb S. As these rare mutations are not targeted in the protocol, only the sickle mutation will be detected, giving screening results that mimic that of a sickle carrier. Examples include Hb Maputo and Hb North Shore.

An update and three-year review of the Welsh screening programme was published in 2017 [8]. At the time of writing, 100,456 babies had been screened using the protocol. Findings were similar to those of previous studies (10 true-positive sickle cell disease cases and 6 false positives) with no false negatives reported. The latter six cases were sickle cell carriers with results that fell above the action value in the Welsh Programme, which aims to detect only sickle cell disease. Such cases are considered to be false positives. The protocol had been transferred successfully to a second instrument maintaining the set action values, which correlated well with values established by the Public Health England (PHE) Sickle Cell & Thalassaemia screening programme [9]. Work had also been carried out to correlate observed ratios of the γ and β chain ratios to gestational age in premature samples and to age after birth. These ratios were used to guide interpretation of results obtained and to reduce the number of samples referred unnecessarily for second testing.

This work was overlapped by a multi-centre pilot study carried out by the PHE Sickle Cell & Thalassaemia screening programme during 2012 and 2013 [10,11]. The aim of the study was to investigate integration of the SpOtOn Clinical Diagnostics method into routine screening services, determine if common action values could be established for all manufacturers and laboratories, and assess consistency with existing methods. Four laboratories participated in the study; 23,878 samples were analysed using either ABI Sciex AP4000 (2 laboratories) or Waters Micromass (Xevo TQMS (1 laboratory) and Premier (1 laboratory) instruments. The study was unable to recommend the use of the latter instrument in this context, as false-positive rates were unacceptably high due to variable ratios. The need to replicate existing practice and ensure consistency with existing methods (HPLC, capillary electrophoresis (CE), and IEF) required the detection of carriers of the targeted haemoglobin variants as well as beta thalassaemia disease. Common action values were set for all experiments with the exception of Hb C, which has manufacturer-specific values [9].

The programme operates a two-test protocol such that results are only reported following second testing, so conservative action values were set to minimise the likelihood of false-negative results from the first line test. The action values are available online [9] and subject to ongoing review and optimisation with laboratories who have implemented the method. At the time of writing, three English newborn screening laboratories have implemented the protocol with a further three actively assessing the method. Over 150 positive cases have been identified in a cohort of approximately 250,000 babies.

The protocol has also been investigated for use in a German setting with 29,079 newborn samples screened as part of an evaluation project carried out between November 2015 and September 2016 in Berlin [12]. Samples were analysed in parallel with CE, with 100% concordance reported. Samples positive for sickle cell disease ($n = 7$) were also confirmed by molecular techniques. The authors have concluded that MSMS is a suitable technique for newborn screening in Germany, citing the benefits of the existing expertise in MSMS techniques as well as the ability to use software algorithms to only find sickle cell disease cases. This is in keeping with the requirements of their genetic testing act, which prohibits the testing of minors for heterozygous states considered to be not relevant in childhood or adolescence [12].

4. Summary

The development of ESI-MSMS for newborn sickle cell disease screening was driven by the concept that rationalization of resource within newborn screening laboratories would be of benefit in a health care environment where there is increasing pressure on equipment, cost, and workforce skill mix. The protocol uses the same equipment as that used for newborn metabolic screening. Initial set up is more time-consuming when compared to HPLC, and is similar to IEF, however analysis and result interpretation time is significantly reduced, particularly if software algorithms are used to scrutinize the data. This also has the advantage of removing operator-dependent variability. The method is targeted and more specific than existing procedures, whilst the inherent flexibility has enabled users to develop protocols that fit with local practice and requirements. Reported sensitivity for Hb S is 100%, where this data is presented [4,11,12]. Costs vary according to laboratory arrangements but are comparable with other available techniques.

Since the first report of the procedure in 2005 [3], the literature shows that the protocol has been adopted in a number of different settings, and it is estimated that more than one million babies have been screened with no false-negative cases reported. The ability to prevent the operator from identifying the majority of cases of carriers fulfils ethical requirements and is seen as advantageous by some users, although use of the protocol in this way does mean that some rare cases of sickle cell disease will be missed. The rationalization of equipment and skills, along with reduced interpretative requirements, is also advantageous in the current environment. Where screening programmes already exist, it is important to ensure standardization with existing practice, and this has been demonstrated to be possible in the English setting [10]. The current lack of an experiment to detect Hb Bart's may limit uptake in areas where this currently falls into newborn screening requirements. However, strategies to target Hb Bart's are being investigated by the manufacturer. Other areas under development include quality control material.

In conclusion, ESI-MSMS has been shown to be a specific, sensitive, and practical technique for newborn screening for sickle cell disease.

5. Patents

WO2006082389A1, Screening method. WO2008/0135756A1, Peptide Standards.

Conflicts of Interest: Charles Turner is a director and shareholder of SpOtOn Clinical Diagnostics. Yvonne Daniel is named as co-inventor on the screening method patent.

References

1. Kiernan, U.A.; Black, J.A.; Williams, P.; Nelson, R.W. High-Throughput analysis of haemoglobin from neonates using matrix-assisted laser desorption/ionization time-of-flight mass spectrometry. *Clin. Chem.* **2002**, *48*, 946–949.
2. Wild, B.J.; Green, B.N.; Stephens, A.D. The potential of electrospray ionization mass spectrometry for the diagnosis of hemoglobin variants found in newborn screening. *Blood Cells Mol. Dis.* **2004**, *33*, 308–317. [CrossRef] [PubMed]
3. Daniel, Y.A.; Turner, C.; Haynes, R.M.; Hunt, B.J.; Dalton, R.N. Rapid and specific detection of clinically significant haemoglobinopathies using electrospray mass spectrometry-mass spectrometry. *Br. J. Haem.* **2005**, *130*, 635–643. [CrossRef] [PubMed]
4. Daniel, Y.; Turner, C.; Farrar, L.; Dalton, R.N. A comparison of IEF and MSMS for clinical hemoglobinopathy screening in 40,000 newborns. *Blood* **2008**, *112*, 2387.
5. Boemer, F.; Ketelslegers, O.; Minon, J.-M.; Bours, V.; Schoos, R. Newborn screening for sickle cell disease using tandem mass spectrometry. *Clin. Chem.* **2008**, *54*, 2036–2041. [CrossRef] [PubMed]
6. Boemer, F.; Cornet, Y.; Libioulle, C.; Segers, K.; Bours, V.; Schoos, R. 3-years experience review of neonatal screening for hemoglobin disorders using tandem mass spectrometry. *Clin. Chim. Act.* **2011**, *412*, 1476–1479. [CrossRef] [PubMed]
7. Moat, S.J.; Rees, D.; King, L.; Ifederu, A.; Harvey, K.; Hall, K.; Lloyd, G.; Morell, G.; Hillier, S. Newborn blood spot screening for sickle cell disease by using tandem mass spectrometry: implementation of a protocol to identify only the disease states of sickle cell disease. *Clin. Chem.* **2014**, *60*, 373–380. [CrossRef] [PubMed]
8. Moat, S.J.; Rees, D.; George, R.S.; King, L.; Dodd, A.; Ifederu, A.; Ramgoolam, T.; Hillier, S. Newborn screening for sickle cell disorders using tandem mass spectrometry: Three years' experience of using a protocol to detect only the disease states. *Ann. Clin. Biochem.* **2017**, *54*, 601–611. [PubMed]
9. Daniel, Y.; Henthorn, J. Public Health England. Available online: https://assets.publishing.service.gov.uk/government/uploads/system/uploads/attachment_data/file/664932/Sickle_cell_and_thalassaemia_screening_action_values_for_tandem_mass_spectrometry_screening.pdf (accessed on 23 November 2018).
10. Daniel, Y.; Henthorn, J. Public Health England. Available online: https://assets.publishing.service.gov.uk/government/uploads/system/uploads/attachment_data/file/488858/Tandem_Mass_Spectrometry_for_Sickle_Cell_and_Thalassaemia_Newborn_Screening_Pilot_Study_2015.pdf (accessed on 23 November 2018).
11. Daniel, Y.A.; Henthorn, J. Newborn screening for sickling and other haemoglobin disorders using tandem mass spectrometry: A pilot study of methodology in laboratories in England. *J. Med. Screen.* **2016**, *23*, 175–178. [CrossRef] [PubMed]
12. Lobitz, S.; Klein, J.; Brose, A.; Blankenstein, O.; Frömmel, C. Newborn screening by tandem mass spectromety confirms the high prevalence of sickle cell disease among German newborns. *Ann. Hem.* **2018**. [CrossRef]

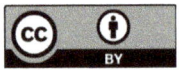

© 2018 by the authors. Licensee MDPI, Basel, Switzerland. This article is an open access article distributed under the terms and conditions of the Creative Commons Attribution (CC BY) license (http://creativecommons.org/licenses/by/4.0/).

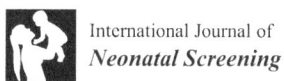

Article

A Multicentre Pilot Study of a Two-Tier Newborn Sickle Cell Disease Screening Procedure with a First Tier Based on a Fully Automated MALDI-TOF MS Platform

Pierre Naubourg [1], Marven El Osta [1], David Rageot [2], Olivier Grunewald [3], Gilles Renom [3], Patrick Ducoroy [1] and Jean-Marc Périni [3,*]

[1] Biomaneo, 22B boulevard Winston Churchill, F-21000 Dijon, France; pierre.naubourg@biomaneo.com (P.N.); marven.elosta@biomaneo.com (M.E.O.); patrick.ducoroy@biomaneo.com (P.D.)
[2] CLIPP, Clinical Innovation Proteomic Platform, Université de Bourgogne Franche Comté, F-21000 Dijon, France; david.rageot@clipproteomic.fr
[3] Newborn Screening Laboratory, Biology and Pathology Center, Lille University Medical Centre, F-59000 Lille, France; olivier.grunewald@chru-lille.fr (O.G.); gilles.renom@chru-lille.fr (G.R.)
* Correspondence: jean-marc.perini@chru-lille.fr

Received: 4 December 2018; Accepted: 21 January 2019; Published: 23 January 2019

Abstract: The reference methods used for sickle cell disease (SCD) screening usually include two analytical steps: a first tier for differentiating haemoglobin S (HbS) heterozygotes, HbS homozygotes and β-thalassemia from other samples, and a confirmatory second tier. Here, we evaluated a first-tier approach based on a fully automated matrix-assisted laser desorption/ionization time-of-flight mass spectrometry (MALDI-TOF MS) platform with automated sample processing, a laboratory information management system and NeoSickle® software for automatic data interpretation. A total of 6701 samples (with high proportions of phenotypes homozygous (FS) or heterozygous (FAS) for the inherited genes for sickle haemoglobin and samples from premature newborns) were screened. The NeoSickle® software correctly classified 98.8% of the samples. This specific blood sample collection was enriched in qualified difficult samples (premature newborns, FAS samples, late and very late samples, etc.). In this study, the sensitivity of FS sample detection was found to be 100% on the Lille MS facility and 99% on the Dijon MS facility, and the specificity of FS sample detection was found to be 100% on both MS facilities. The MALDI-MS platform appears to be a robust solution for first-tier use to detect the HbS variant: it is reproducible and sensitive, it has the power to analyze 600–1000 samples per day and it can reduce the unit cost of testing thanks to maximal automation, minimal intervention by the medical team and good overall practicability. The MALDI-MS approach meets today's criteria for the large-scale, cost-effective screening of newborns, children and adults.

Keywords: newborn screening; sickle cell disease; MALDI-TOF; mass spectrometry; thalassemia; prevention

1. Introduction

The use of mass spectrometry (MS) to screen newborns for haemoglobinopathies differs from the MS-based diagnosis of a broad range of clinically significant haemoglobin (Hb) variants. Newborn screening requires a robust, high-throughput and cost-effective MS method that solely detects the biomarkers of sickle cell disease (SCD) and β-thalassemia major. In contrast, the broader diagnostic procedure involves the detection of as many changes in globin proteins as possible in a single step. Newborn screening programs are typically organised as single-tier or two-tier procedures. In the two-tier procedure, the first tier is typically a routine MS method (electrospray ionization

(ESI)-MS [1–3] or matrix-assisted laser desorption/ionization (MALDI)-MS [4,5] capable of analysing intact globin chains. Pathological samples with a single mutation in the Hb β-chain can thus be unambiguously classified into three groups: heterozygotes without HbS variants, heterozygotes with HbS variants and HbS homozygotes [5]. Furthermore, β-globin production defects (β-thalassemia) can be detected [5]. The second tier is based on standard methods (such as HPLC, isoelectric focusing, and capillary electrophoresis (CE)) in order to distinguish between heterozygotes Hb F/AS (FAS) and compound heterozygotes (F/SC, F/SD, F/SE and F/S-OArab). In a single-tier procedure, only the most common variants (e.g., HbS, HbC, D^{Punjab}, OArab and HbE) are detected in a tryptic peptide analysis of haemoglobin using ESI-MS/MS [4,6–8] or the direct surface sampling of dried blood spots coupled to high-resolution MS [9–11].

In a multicentre pilot study, we evaluated a two-tier newborn SCD screening procedure in which the first tier is based on the fully automated MALDI-TOF MS classification of Hb profiles as FA, FS or FAS. To achieve this "plug-and-play" first tier, we maximised the performance levels of our previously described preanalytical and analytical procedures [5]. Likewise, we improved the software used for automatic data interpretation. Lastly, a laboratory information management system was set up to ensure data traceability. We investigated the usability of this MALDI-TOF MS newborn SCD screening platform by assessing its analytical throughput, user-friendliness, ease of implementation, potential interfering factors, MS spectral quality and percentage of correctly classified samples. We established quality criteria for standard and nonstandard MS profiles as a function of the newborn's phenotype, determined our algorithm's ability to correctly classify MS profiles and identified interfering factors and their causes. Lastly, we performed a preliminary analysis of the impact of β chain variants other than HbS on the MALDI-TOF profile. Newborns having received one or more blood transfusions were excluded from the present analysis, and are being assessed in a separate, dedicated study. Our results demonstrated the potential value of a MALDI-TOF MS approach for high-throughput newborn SCD screening.

2. Materials and Methods

2.1. Sample Collection

Residual blood spots from standard Guthrie cards (used in our laboratory's routine screening activity) were investigated with MALDI-TOF MS. All samples were collected with the parents' consent for use in the French national newborn screening programme. No additional consent was required because the specimens were not used for purposes other than for which the blood sample was initially collected. The source of the samples has been described previously [5]. The study was registered with the French National Consultative Committee on Information Processing in Medical Research (*Comité consultatif sur le traitement de l'Information en matière de recherche dans le domaine de la santé*; reference: 14.818 12/23/2014). After collection, the samples were anonymised and stored at +4 °C.

Sets of samples from our routine activity were selected each week, according to the following criteria: (i) samples presenting a β chain variant in CE and HPLC assays; (ii) samples from premature newborns (gestational age at delivery: 22–32 weeks); (iii) samples corresponding to late and very late screening; and (iv) and randomly selected samples of daily screening activity that had an interpretable CE profile.

We analyzed 6701 samples with full datasets (i.e., with clinical data as follows: N° of sample, sex, term, weight, name of maternity, transfusion, maternity location and date of screening, birth date plus validated results using CE in the first line and HPLC in the second line; Table 1). The percentage of FAS and FS phenotypes was higher for the premature newborns than for a standard population of newborns. The sample collection date was optimal (3–5 days after delivery) for the great majority of newborns.

Table 1. Characteristics of the newborns and samples.

Phenotype	Number	Term			Sample Collection Date			
		23–32 weeks	33–36 weeks	>37 weeks	3–5 day	6–10 day	11–30 day	>30 day
FS	71	0	5	66	67	3	1	0
F/A	2834	203	809	1822	2651	90	77	16
F/AC	576	13	50	513	547	20	2	7
F/AE	141	2	9	130	138	2	0	1
F/AO-Arab	21	0	2	19	19	2	0	0
F/AD	17	0	0	17	17	0	0	0
F/AKorle-Bu	10	0	0	10	10	0	0	0
F/AX	86	4	3	79	81	3	0	2
F/C	7	0	1	6	6	0	0	1
F/E	3	0	0	3	2	1	0	0
F/O-Arab	1	0	0	1	1	0	0	0
Corrected FA	3696	222	874	2600	3472	118	79	
F/AS	2894	57	247	2590	2763	89	23	19
F/SC	23	0	1	22	22	1	0	0
F/SE	1	0	0	1	1	0	0	0
F/SO-Arab	1	0	1	0	1	0	0	0
Corrected FAS	2919	57	249	2613	2787	90	23	19
S-β^+-thalassaemia	15	0	1	14	15	0	0	0

The number of corrected FA phenotype corresponding to the sum of all samples (FA, FAC, FAE, FAO-Arab, FAD, FAKorle-Bu, FAX, FC, FE, FO Arab where either β^A gene was duplicated [$\beta^A\beta^A$] or associated with other β chain variants ($\beta^A\beta^C$, $\beta^A\beta^E$, $\beta^A\beta^{O\text{-}Arab}$, $\beta^A\beta^D$, $\beta^A\beta^C$, $\beta^A\beta^X$) or where duplicate ß chain variants were found ($\beta^C\beta^C$, $\beta^E\beta^E$, $\beta^{O\text{ }Arab}\beta^{O\text{-}Arab}$) that are detected FA by MALDI. The number of corrected FAS phenotype corresponding to the sum of all heterozygous (FAS) and composite heterozygous (FSC, FSE, FSO-Arab) samples where βS gene was associated respectively to βA gene or to other ß chain variants ($\beta^S\beta^C$, $\beta^S\beta^E$, $\beta^S\beta^{O\text{-}Arab}$) that are detected FAS by MALDI.

2.2. Definition of Corrected Phenotypes

Subjects who were heterozygous or homozygous for HbC, HbD-Punjab, HbE, HbO-Arab, HbKorle-Bu and some unidentified variants (HbX) according to conventional methods were detected as HbA by linear MALDI-TOF due to the technique's lack of mass resolution. Hence, these newborns were classified as having a corrected FA phenotype. Likewise, corrected FAS phenotypes included the composite heterozygous FSC, FSE and FS-OArab phenotypes.

2.3. Sample Processing and Analysis

In the present pilot study, all samples were measured with MALDI-MS at two analytical facilities (the University of Burgundy's CLIPP facility (Dijon, France) and Lille University Hospital's newborn screening laboratory (Lille, France)) after two chips (diameter: 3.5 mm) had been isolated from each blood spot.

2.4. Sample Preparation for MS Measurements

At both facilities, samples were prepared for MS measurements using a research version of the NeoSickle® kit (Biomaneo, Dijon, France) for an EVO 200 automated system in Dijon and an EVO 100 automated system in Lille (Tecan, Lyon, France). The NeoSickle® kit was used according to the manufacturer's instructions, which included a first step of solubilization of proteins by a specific solution, and a second step of mixing with the matrix that was specially adapted for the MALDI-TOF MS analysis of blood proteins. The sample–matrix mixture was then deposited in quadruplicate on a 384-spot polished steel MALDI target (Bruker Daltonik GmbH, Bremen, Germany).

2.5. Mass Spectrometry Measurements

At both facilities, MS was performed with a MALDI-TOF system (an AutoFlex™ Speed with a 2000 Hz Smartbeam™ II laser (Bruker Daltonik GmbH) in Dijon, and an AutoFlex™ III with a 200 Hz Smartbeam™ laser (Bruker Daltonik GmbH) in Lille.

2.6. Data Processing

Mass spectrometry acquisitions were analyzed by the algorithm if (i) the whole spectrum and the region of interest were sufficiently intense, (ii) the baseline was not too noisy and (iii) at least three of the four profiles per sample could be interpreted automatically. After evaluation of the quality of each spectrum, the spectra were normalized, smoothed and underwent baseline subtraction. The four spectra obtained of the same sample were then averaged to obtain a mean profile, which was submitted to the algorithm.

2.7. Analytical Data Flow

An algorithm for automatic discrimination between normal samples and samples containing an HbS variant had been developed using spectra from an initial cohort of phenotyped samples by CE and HPLC. It has since been improved as further data are acquired. All of the analytical results were centralized via a secure data collector and submitted to the algorithm. The median newborns' profiles were automatically classified as FA, FAS or FS.

2.8. Visual Assessment of MS Profiles

In order to evaluate the algorithm's ability to classify a newborn's profile as FA, FAS or FS, all of the following profiles were visually inspected: (i) samples classified as FS or FAS by CE/HPLC, (ii) samples for which MALDI-MS and CE/HPLC gave conflicting results, (iii) samples with abnormal CE and/or HPLC profiles, (iv) samples from premature newborns, (v) samples with β chain variants other than HbS, (vi) samples with low-intensity MS signals at 15,850 m/z and 15,880 m/z [5], (vii) samples with a "low HbA" warning and (viii) samples for which the Dijon and Lille facilities gave conflicting results. Lastly, half the remaining samples (classified as FA by both HPLC and CE) were checked at random.

2.9. The Data Collector

Sickle Cell Anemia Collect & Compare (SCACC) is a web application developed by Biomaneo to help biologists compare MS screening results with those of the reference screening methods (CE and HPLC). Within a single application, SCACC can store, group and present heterogeneous data in a user-friendly way, including clinical data on the sample donor, the experimental data from CE and HPLC analyses, the experimental data from the MS analysis and the validation files (i.e., the screening results sent to the paediatrician).

The SCACC application contains a table in which all of the information available for a given sample is shown on a single line. Along with a filter system for each variable, this layout makes it easy to create pools of interest (preterm samples, pathologic results, etc.) for the analysis of any misinterpreted results.

3. Results

3.1. Optimization of Preanalytical and Analytical Procedures

In France, newborn SCD screening is centralized at a few specialist analytical centres. This centralisation requires a very-high-throughput system capable of analyzing 600–1000 samples per day. The MALDI-TOF MS approach meets this requirement: for each run, it takes 1 h to deposit 288 samples in quadruplicate on three 384-spot MALDI targets.

Using an AutoFlex™ Speed system, it took 22 min to analyze a MALDI target containing 96 samples. Hence, the analytical throughput was estimated to be around 210 samples/hour; it took 5 h to analyze 1056 samples.

One of the essential criteria for automation was easy operation of the software that controlled the platform and displayed the results. A technician with little experience of MS could perform analyses on the MALDI-TOF MS system interfaced with the workstation. Another strong point is that all of the data from an analytical run were published and aggregated into a 96-well plate format. Abnormal profiles were differentiated from normal profiles by a colour code. Three different icons can be showed within a given coloured square: a cross indicating that the profile could not be interpreted, an exclamation mark indicating that the profile's initial automatic classification has been modified manually or a question mark indicating that the profile did not match the phenotype and must be checked by the operator. The spectrum's region of interest can be displayed in a mode in which β, βS and γ chains are seen or in a zoom mode in which only the β and βS chains are seen (Figure 1). The abnormal MS profiles were assessed visually by the operator. When applicable, two decision-support warnings could be displayed by the algorithm: "low HbA concentration" or "newborn having received a blood transfusion". The data for a given newborn (ID number, demographic data, zoom mode or not, classification changes and non-hidden alerts) can be displayed by clicking on a well.

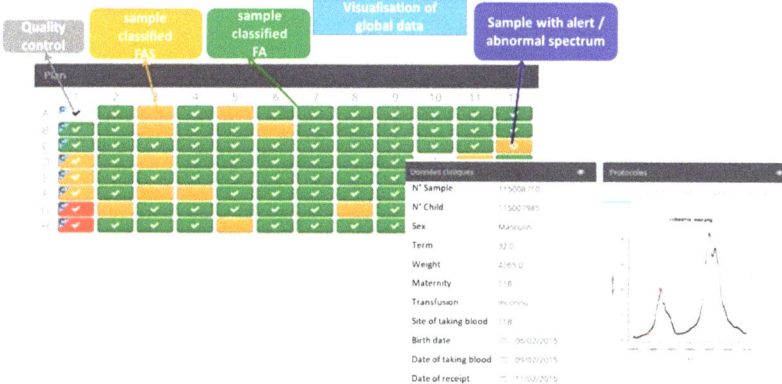

Figure 1. A screen display from the Sickle Cell Anemia Collect & Compare (SCACC) web application. Each box corresponds to a position of a sample on the 96-well plate. The green box corresponds to one sample classified FA, the orange box corresponds to one sample classified FAS and the red boxes are samples detected as FS. The software presents on the same page the clinical data (N° of sample, sex, term, weight, name of maternity, transfusion, location and date of taking blood, birth date) and the spectra of one sample.

3.2. Spectral Quality of MALDI-TOF Data

Taken as a whole, our results show NeoSickle®'s ability to correctly classify 97% of the samples tested in Lille and 98.8% of the samples tested in Dijon. The sensitivity of the NeoSickle® approaches to detect the FA samples is 99.2% and 97.2% with a specificity of 99% and 99.3% on the Lille and the Dijon MS facility, respectively. The detection of an HbS chain in samples is obtained on the Lille and the Dijon MS facility with a sensitivity of 98.4% and 97% and with a specificity of 99.8% and 99%, respectively.

The positive predictive value of FS profiles detection was 96.6% and 97.7% with the results obtained by the Lille and the Dijon MS facility, respectively. The negative predictive value of FS profiles detection obtained at Lille and the Dijon MS facility was 100% and 99.9%, respectively.

It is important to note that these results were obtained with biased blood samples that were enriched in FS and FAS samples and difficult samples (premature newborns, very late screening).

3.2.1. Criteria Used to Define a Standard MALDI-TOF Profile

In 85.8% of the analyses in Dijon and 92.9% of the analyses in Lille, the median FA, FAS, FS and S-β$^+$ MS profiles (Figure 2a,c,e,g, respectively) were considered to be standard and were automatically interpreted by the NeoSickle® software. Limits not to be exceeded were defined: an FA profile with a low-noise ascending or convex baseline was considered to be normal (Figure 2b); an FAS profile was considered to be standard as long as a plateau separated the β^S and β^A chain peaks (Figure 2d);

and, lastly, an FS profile with a low-noise ascending or convex baseline to the right of the β^S chain peak was considered to be interpretable (Figure 2f). The profile of a newborn with S-β^+-thalassemia was characterized by a much more intense β^S peak, relative to the β^A peak (Figure 2g,h).

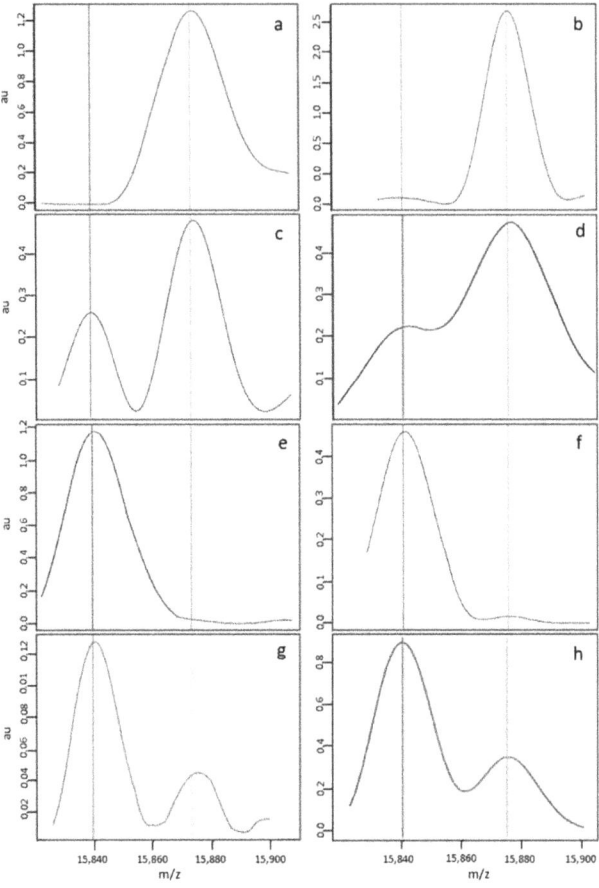

Figure 2. Examples of standard MS profiles correctly classified by the NeoSickle® software, from newborns with the following phenotypes: FA (**a,b**), FAS (**c,d**), FS (**e,f**) and S-β + (**g,h**).

3.2.2. Classification by the Algorithm of "Standard" Profiles, as a Function of the Newborn's Corrected Phenotype

There were no classification errors among the corrected FA and FS samples (Table 2). Concerning the corrected FAS samples, only 2 of the 2753 standard profiles from Lille were misclassified (as FS) by MS, and 17 of the 2507 standard profiles from Dijon were misclassified (16 cases classified as FA by MS, and 1 case classified as FS by MS). Although the spectra of the FAS samples misclassified as FA showed a shoulder with a plateau at 15,850 $m/z \pm 10$ m/z, the signal intensity was too low. This characteristic should be introduced in the criteria for a nonstandard MS profile.

The FAS samples misclassified as FS by MALDI-MS came from composite heterozygous newborns classified as FS-O Arab and FSE by CE and HPLC. Regular peaks at 18,850 and 1880 m/z were observed; however, the error was induced by the low intensity of the peak at 15,880 m/z. A profile with asymmetry for the β^A and β^S chains (a more intense β^S peak) prompted its classification as FS by the e-NeoSickle software.

Table 2. The number of standard MS profiles correctly classified (+) or misclassified (−), according to the newborn's corrected phenotype.

	Lille MS Facility						Dijon MS Facility					
Number of Standard Profiles	6181						5698					
Corrected Phenotype	FA		FAS		FS		FA		FAS		FS	
Number of samples	3386		2753		37		3161		2507		35	
classification by the algorithm	+	−	+	−	+	−	+	−	+	−	+	−
	3386	0	2751	2	37	0	3161	0	2490	17	35	0

The 16 samples misclassified in Dijon gave good results in Lille, indicating that the errors were probably due to a temporary lack of spectrum quality and not a sample or detection problem. The quality of the Dijon data was not as high as in Lille because the number of nonstandard spectra was higher; this finding agrees with the higher misclassification rate observed in Dijon.

3.2.3. Description of a Nonstandard MALDI-MS Profile

A nonstandard median MS profile was detected in 14.7% of the analyses in Dijon and 7.6% of the analyses in Lille. The MS profiles were considered to be nonstandard (Figure 3) for one of three reasons. Firstly (cause 1, see Table 3), some profiles had a nonregular baseline or a slightly distorted peak; this applied to (i) FA MS profiles with a variably broad/sharp/distorted peak but very low intensity at 15,837 $m/z \pm 5$ Da, relative to the β^A peak (Figure 3a,b); an FAS MS profile with minor deformation of the β^S peak (Figure 3c); and FS and S-β^+-thalassemia MS profiles with an irregular baseline (data not shown) and a deformation of the β^A peak (Figure 3d). Secondly (cause 2), some profiles had a low, broad peak at 15,837 m/z; this applied to (i) FA MS profiles with a variably shifted peak or (ii) FAS MS profiles characterized by a broad, well-centred peak at 15,837 ± 5 m/z but that was much less intense than the β^A chain peak at 15,867 m/z (data not shown). Thirdly (cause 3), some FA MS profiles had a broader β^A peak that variably overlapped with the region of interest at 15,837 m/z and led to misclassification as "FAS" (Figure 3e), whereas other FAS MS profiles showed a low resolution and thus poor separation of the β^A and β^S peaks, giving a single large peak as a shoulder and no plateau between the peaks (Figure 3f).

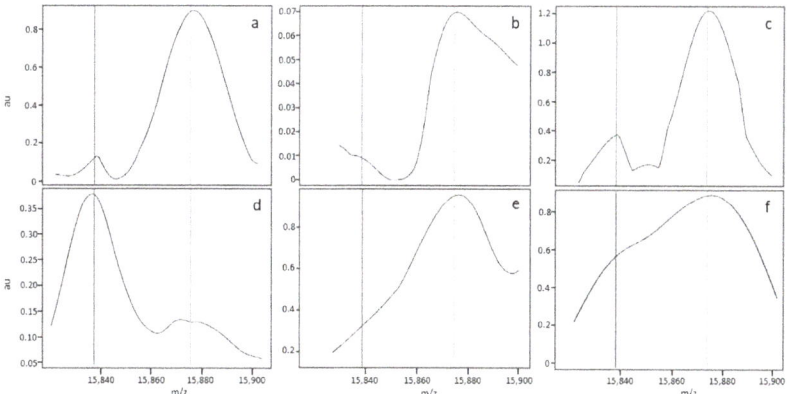

Figure 3. Zoom of MS profiles on the zone of interest for nonstandard FA (**a,b,e**), FAS (**c,f**) and FS (**d**) samples.

3.2.4. Classification by the Algorithm of Profiles Considered to be Nonstandard in a Visual Assessment, as a Function of the Newborn's Corrected Phenotype

The data in Table 3 show that the great majority of nonstandard profiles (84.5% in Lille and 81.2% in Dijon) were nevertheless correctly classified by the e-NeoSickle® algorithm. Furthermore, 7.5% of the nonstandard profiles in Lille and 4.6% of the nonstandard profiles Dijon were misclassified, and 8% of the nonstandard profiles in Lille and 14.2% of the nonstandard profiles in Dijon were uninterpretable.

It is important to note that the nonstandard profiles accounted for less than 14% of the analyses in Dijon and 7% of the analyses in Lille. Overall, only 2% of the profiles in Dijon and 0.6% of the profiles in Lille were uninterpretable, and 0.9% of the profiles in Dijon and 0.6% of the profiles in Lille were misclassified.

Table 3. Classification by the algorithm of profiles considered to be nonstandard in a visual assessment. Some spectra could not be interpreted by the algorithm (IN). The percentage is based on the number of profiles considered to be nonstandard (780 profiles at Lille and 985 at Dijon).

			Corrected Phenotypes		
			FA	FAS	FS
MALDI-TOF MS classification of non-standard profiles	Lille	FA	282 (54.7%)	30 (5.9%)	0 (0%)
		FAS	7 (1.4%)	118 (23.2%)	0 (0%)
		FS	0 (0%)	1 (0.2%)	34 (6.7%)
		IN	21 (4.5%)	17 (3.4%)	0 (0%)
	Dijon	FA	446 (45%)	22 (2.2%)	0 (0%)
		FAS	21 (2.2%)	323 (32.7%)	1 (0.2%)
		FS	0 (0%)	1 (0.2%)	36 (3.7%)
		IN	68 (7.2%)	67 (6.8%)	0 (0%)

The frequencies of "nonregular baseline" (cause 1) and "low/broad peak" (cause 2) features were similar at the two MS facilities. Our analysis showed that most of the nonstandard spectra in Dijon (54%) were due to a lack of resolution (cause 3), whereas this was the case for only 13% in Lille. Proportionally, the corrected phenotype FS ($n = 71$) was more likely to be labelled as "low resolution", with respectively 31 and 36 abnormal spectra in Lille and Dijon. However, this low resolution had very little impact on the automatic classification, since less than 1% of all spectra labelled as "low resolution" were misclassified.

Sixteen percent of the spectra with a low, broad peak at 15,837 m/z were misclassified by the algorithm (Table 4). Of the 21 spectra of this type misclassified in Lille, 20 (95%) came from newborns with a corrected FAS phenotype. Likewise, of the 20 spectra of this type misclassified in Dijon (Table 4), 18 (90%) came from newborns with a corrected FAS phenotype. These spectra were very difficult to classify because the ratio between the β^S and β^A peaks was abnormal. A very low β^S peak (relative to the β^A peak) can be interpreted as a sample with high background noise or as a sample from an S homozygote or an AS heterozygote having received a blood transfusion (which induces a strong imbalance). Given that these spectra have low peak intensities, we recommend repeating the analysis or depositing a new sample.

Table 4. (A) Numbers and proportions of nonstandard spectra by corrected phenotype and by cause. (B) Numbers and proportions of correctly classified and misclassified spectra by cause. Cause 1 resulted in spectra with an irregular baseline, cause 2 resulted in spectra with a low, broad peak and cause 3 resulted in spectra with a low resolution. The percentage is based on the number of profiles considered to be nonstandard (780 profiles at Lille and 985 at Dijon).

A		Corrected Phenoztype			B		Correctly Classified	Misclassified
		FA	FAS	FS				
Lille	Cause 1	179 (37%)	90 (19%)	3 (0%)	Lille	Cause 1	252 (94%)	17 (6%)
	Cause 2	98 (21%)	28 (5%)	0 (0%)		Cause 2	105 (84%)	21 (16%)
	Cause 3	12 (3%)	31 (7%)	31 (7%)		Cause 3	77 (100%)	0 (0%)
Dijon	Cause 1	193 (23%)	69 (8%)	0 (0%)	Dijon	Cause 1	248 (95%)	14 (5%)
	Cause 2	103 (12%)	24 (3%)	0 (0%)		Cause 2	107 (84%)	20 (16%)
	Cause 3	171 (20%)	253 (30%)	36 (4%)		Cause 3	449 (98%)	11 (2%)

3.2.5. Causes of Abnormal Spectral Features in Nonstandard MS Profiles

A spectral analysis showed that nonstandard profiles mainly resulted from the compilation of differing spectra within a quadruplicate. Figure 4 shows the variability in the raw data and its impact on data processing. The spectra in Figure 4a,b,e,f correspond to the raw data generated for the first (Figure 4a,b) and third (Figure 4e,f) of the quadruplicate sample depositions. The two depositions varied markedly in terms of the raw spectral intensity (less than 40 ua for deposition 1, and 200 ua for deposition 3). The data processing steps (including peak alignment and baseline normalisation and subtraction) normalise the spectrum intensity but also remove differences (see Figure 4c,g, corresponding to the normalized spectra, and a blow-up view of the zone of interest Figure 4d,h). The compilation of normalized data introduces a bias, and might lead to misinterpretation of the results by the software. Figure 4i shows a median spectrum with an irregular baseline; this "pseudo β^S peak" can be confused with a true β^S peak. However, the relative intensity of the pseudo β^S peak differed from that of a true β^A peak.

The analysis of each individual spectrum enabled us to affirm that at least one good-quality, high-resolution spectrum was obtained for each biological sample. The sample deposition method for MALDI-MS is known not to be highly reproducible, and thus makes it difficult to obtain very homogeneous results. Even though our study highlighted this difficulty, our analysis also showed that a high-quality result can be obtained systematically.

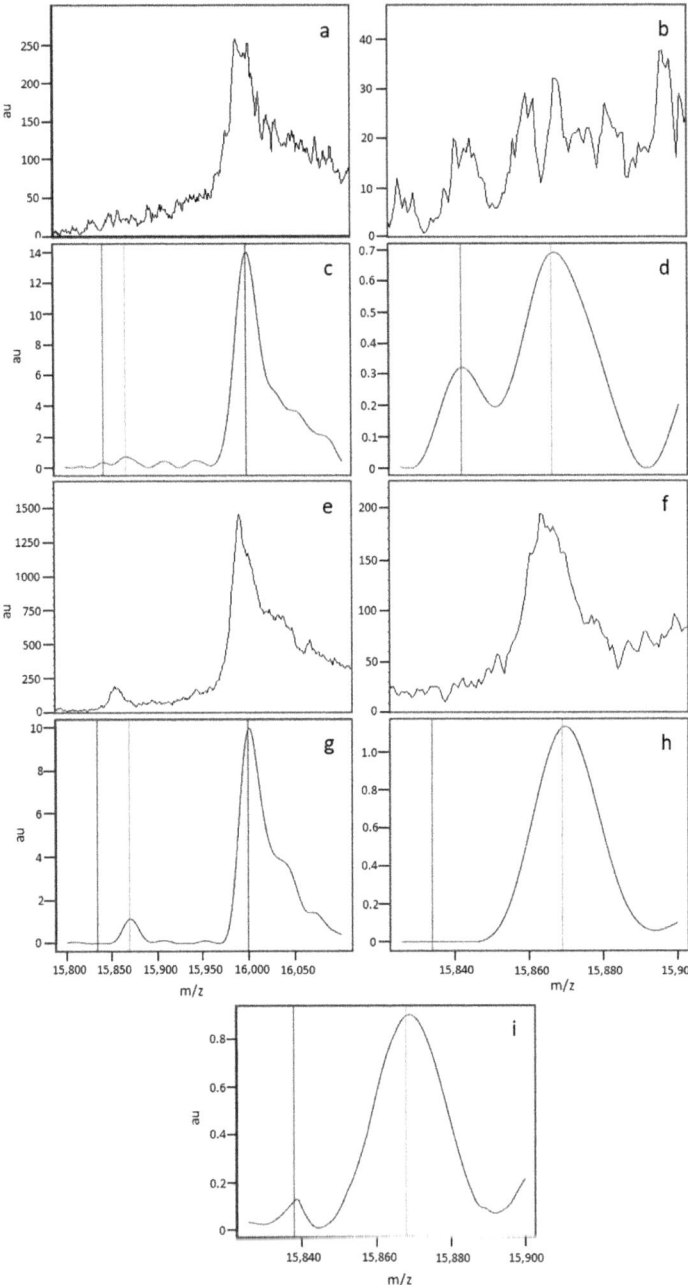

Figure 4. The spectra in (a,b,e,f) correspond to the raw data generated for the first (a,b) and third (e,f) of the quadruplicate depositions from the same sample. (a,c,e,g) show the whole spectrum (15,800–16,100 Da), and (b–f,h,i) show the region of interest (15,820–15,900 Da). The spectra in (c–h correspond to the processed spectra after alignment, baseline subtraction, and normalisation. The median spectrum (i) was obtained by compiling the individual normalized spectra.

4. Occasional Misclassifications

The analysis of samples that were classified differently by the two analytical facilities confirmed that MALDI-MS can provide an interpretable result for each sample. In fact, the data in Table 5 showed that the 68 samples with a corrected FA phenotype that could not be interpreted in Dijon were correctly classified in Lille (67 standard spectra and 1 low-resolution spectrum). Likewise, the 21 samples with a corrected FA phenotype and that could not be interpreted in Lille were correctly classified at Dijon. Identical results were obtained with the corrected FAS samples.

Table 5. Paired classification of the samples by the two analytical facilities. Relationship with the spectral quality. This table summarizes the number of profiles correctly classified, misclassified and uninterpretable for each category of profile quality and for the two analytical laboratories.

		\multicolumn{10}{c}{Profile Abnormalities at $15,850 \pm 10$ m/z}									
		\multicolumn{10}{c}{Neonates with a Corrected FA Phenotype}									
Automatic Classification of Matched Profiles		Irregular Base Line		Low, Broad Peak		Low Resolution		Regular Base Line		Uninterpretable	
Lille	Dijon	Lille	Dijon	Lille	Dijon	Lille	Dijon	Lille	Dijon	Lille	Dijon
correctly classified	uninterpretable	1	0	0	0	0	0	67	0	0	68
correctly classified	Misclassified	4	10	7	0	1	5	17	0	0	0
uninterpretable	correctly classified	0	0	0	0	0	0	0	21	0	0
Misclassified	correctly classified	4	0	3	0	0	0	0	7	0	0
		\multicolumn{10}{c}{Neonates with a Corrected FAS Phenotype}									
Automatic Classification of Matched Profiles		Irregular Base Line		Low, Broad Peak		Low Resolution		Regular Base Line		Uninterpretable	
Lille	Dijon	Lille	Dijon	Lille	Dijon	Lille	Dijon	Lille	Dijon	Lille	Dijon
correctly classified	uninterpretable	0	0	0	0	0	0	68	0	0	68
correctly classified	Misclassified	0	4	0	14	1	5	23	0	0	0
uninterpretable	correctly classified	0	0	0	0	0	1	0	16	17	0
Misclassified	correctly classified	12	0	12	0	0	4	6	26	0	0

When a profile was misclassified or uninterpretable at one MS facility, the corresponding profile at the other MS facility was correctly classified and was less likely to be a nonstandard profile. Only one sample with a nonstandard profile was misclassified at both MS facilities (data not shown). A good classification with a standard spectrum was obtained for each sample on at least one of the MS facilities, which indicates that a low HbA concentration was not the main cause of misclassifications or uninterpretable results. Misclassifications or uninterpretable results were mainly due to the absence of a high-quality spectrum induced by technical incidents (tip blockage and non-deposition of the sample). Consequently, repeating the analysis of a sample with a nonstandard profile was the best way of obtaining a standard profile and a correct classification. Different data, such as peak intensities or the ratio between different peaks of β^A and β^S chains, allow for us to detect the nonstandard profile and to add an alert to the results.

5. Discussion

Newborn disease screening programmes are front-line public health measures, and as such must be based on robust analytical methods and data-processing software. Cost effectiveness is a further requirement, prompting the implementation of high-throughput screening units that reduce unit costs. Lastly, the maximal use of automation enables the analytical results to be validated with as little intervention as possible by the medical team. Our MALDI-MS platform and the associated data-processing and interpretation software were designed to address these challenges.

In newborn SCD screening with a MALDI MS system, the user-friendliness of the software interface and a high-throughput analysis coupled to automatic sample classification and traceability are directly related to practicability. As mentioned above, newborn SCD screening in France is centralised at a few specialist analytical centres. This centralisation requires a throughput of up to 600–1000 samples per day. The MALDI-TOF MS approach meets this requirement.

The next performance criterion of note concerns the method's robustness: in other words, its ability to generate good-quality standard MS profiles that enable correct classification in agreement with the sample's validated phenotype, whatever the newborn's clinical status. In order to test our MALDI-MS under extreme conditions, we increased the proportion of difficult samples in the presently analyzed cohort; this corresponds to pathological specimens and specimens collected and/or stored under non-optimal conditions (samples from premature newborns, samples collected long after delivery, samples collected from France's overseas regions and dependencies that may have been stored for a long time in a tropical atmosphere before delivery to the screening laboratory in continental France, etc.). In the present study, only samples from newborns having received one or more blood transfusions were discarded. The impact of blood transfusion will be described in a specific study of the effect of high HbA levels on the method's sensitivity, specificity and resolution as a function of the β^S chain concentration. Moreover, we evaluated the MALDI-TOF method's robustness by visually checking the spectral quality as well as by considering its ability to correctly classify the newborns as FA, FAS or FS. Benchmark MALDI-TOF MS spectra were thus established on the basis of the classification results and the visual quality of the spectra. The reference spectra correspond to all of the spectra defined as standard for which the information obtained is considered to be sufficient and of good quality. Indeed, visual spectral validation has proved to be most effective for revealing shot-to-shot variations.

Using this strategy, we determined the percentages of newborns with a standard profile and who were correctly classified (relative to their validated phenotype). The highest level of efficiency was obtained in the set of newborns with a corrected FA phenotype; around 85% of these analyses could be validated directly. A similar percentage was obtained for newborns with a corrected FAS phenotype. Moreover, nonstandard MS spectra were not systematically misclassified, and most were correctly classified. We consider these results to be very promising because it should be possible to further improve the procedures for sample deposition, raw data analysis and selection of the mass spectra to which the classification algorithm is applied.

None of the samples from FS newborns were misclassified, and a sample with an FAS-corrected phenotype was misclassified as an FA sample. This type of misclassification can lead to false negatives for newborns with an FSC phenotype. This major error required us to set up a strategy for correcting the automatic classification. The development and characteristics of tracking alerts for the nonstandard MS profiles will be described elsewhere. This approach should enable an occasional lack of reproducibility, sensitivity or resolution in Hb profiling to be detected.

There were two main reasons for the incorrect automatic classification of newborn phenotypes. Firstly, a low signal intensity at 15,850 and/or 15,880 m/z (i.e., similar to background noise) was intensified by the data processing (normalisation and alignment). Secondly, poor resolution of the ß and/or β^S chains generated signal overlap. The quadruplicate sample analysis improved the results, but was not always able to counterbalance shot-to-shot variability.

In a previous article [5], very poor spectral quality prevented the analysis of 20 of 844 samples (2.5%), even after several repeat analyses. The relatively high frequency of this incident was probably due to the inclusion of a high proportion of samples from premature newborns and/or HbS carriers. We have now resolved this problem. In most cases, a single repeat analysis was enough to obtain a standard profile. Some problems arose from time to time but were mainly related to robotic preparation of the blood spot samples. Further optimization of sample processing and the MS acquisition protocol should further improve the standardization of the MS profiles and reduce the frequency of repeat analysis.

Taken as a whole, our results for pooled standard and nonstandard spectra demonstrated NeoSickle®'s ability to classify correctly 97% of the samples tested in Lille and 98.8% of the samples tested in Dijon. Furthermore, only 2% of the nonstandard spectra in Dijon were uninterpretable, and less than 0.9% were misclassified. In Lille, 0.6% of the nonstandard spectra were uninterpretable and 0.6% were misclassified. It is important to note that these percentages were obtained with "difficult" blood samples (premature newborns, very late screening).

Our pilot study showed that the NeoSickle® approach can differentiate between heterozygous FSE, FSO-Arab and S-β + samples on one hand and heterozygous FAS and homozygous FS samples on the other. Indeed, the signal intensity of the β^E, β^{O-Arab} variants was much weaker than that of the β chain.

In addition to classifying samples as FA, FAS or FS, studies of a larger cohort of patients might make it possible to clearly differentiate a fourth class (corresponding to heterozygous SX samples in which the β^X chain is E, O-Arab, a).

In conclusion, our new MALDI-TOF MS approach already meets today's requirements [12] for large-scale, cost-effective newborn SCD screening, and is well-positioned to address future requirements for even greater throughputs and total automation to detect the HbS variants.

Author Contributions: D.R. and M.E.O.: MALDI-TOF methodology; P.N.: software development; G.R. and O.G.: validation; P.D. and J.-M.P.: conceptualization, data curation, acquisition of funding and drafting of the manuscript.

Funding: The present research was funded by Lille University Medical Center and the Conseil Régional de Bourgogne.

Conflicts of Interest: Patrick Ducoroy was an employee of the University of Burgundy at the time of the research described here. He then founded the company Biomaneo, and currently serves as its CEO.

References

1. Rai, D.K.; Griffiths, W.J.; Landin, B.; Wild, B.J.; Alvelius, G.; Green, B.N. Accurate mass measurement by electrospray ionization quadrupole mass spectrometry: Detection of variants differing by <6 Da from normal in human hemoglobin heterozygotes. *Anal. Chem.* **2003**, *75*, 1978–1982. [CrossRef] [PubMed]
2. Wild, B.J.; Green, B.N.; Cooper, E.K.; Lalloz, M.R.; Erten, S.; Stephens, A.D.; Layton, D.M. Rapid identification of hemoglobin variants by electrospray ionization mass spectrometry. *Blood Cells Mol. Dis.* **2001**, *27*, 691–704. [CrossRef] [PubMed]
3. Wild, B.J.; Green, B.N.; Stephens, A.D. The potential of electrospray ionization mass spectrometry for the diagnosis of hemoglobin variants found in newborn screening. *Blood Cells Mol. Dis.* **2004**, *33*, 308–317. [CrossRef] [PubMed]
4. Kiernan, U.A.; Black, J.A.; Williams, P.; Nelson, R.W. High-throughput analysis of hemoglobin from neonates using matrix-assisted laser desorption/ionization time-of-flight mass spectrometry. *Clin. Chem.* **2002**, *48*, 947–949. [PubMed]
5. Hachani, J.; Duban-Deweer, S.; Pottiez, G.; Renom, G.; Flahaut, C.; Périni, J.M. MALDI-TOF MS profiling as the first-tier screen for sickle cell disease in neonates: Matching throughput to objectives. *Proteomics Clin. Appl.* **2011**, *5*, 405–414. [CrossRef] [PubMed]
6. Daniel, Y.A.; Turner, C.; Haynes, R.M.; Hunt, B.J.; Dalton, R.N. Rapid and specific detection of clinically significant haemoglobinopathies using electrospray mass spectrometry-mass spectrometry. *Br. J. Haematol.* **2005**, *130*, 635–643. [CrossRef] [PubMed]
7. Boemer, F.; Ketelslegers, O.; Minon, J.M.; Bours, V.; Schoos, R. Newborn screening for sickle cell disease using tandem mass spectrometry. *Clin. Chem.* **2008**, *54*, 2036–2041. [CrossRef] [PubMed]
8. Moat, S.J.; Rees, D.; King, L.; Ifederu, A.; Harvey, K.; Hall, K.; Lloyd, G.; Morrell, C.; Hillier, S. Newborn blood spot screening for sickle cell disease by using tandem mass spectrometry: Implementation of a protocol to identify only the disease states of sickle cell disease. *Clin. Chem.* **2014**, *60*, 373–380. [CrossRef] [PubMed]
9. Edwards, R.L.; Griffiths, P.; Bunch, J.; Cooper, H.J. Compound heterozygotes and beta-thalassemia: Top-down mass spectrometry for detection of hemoglobinopathies. *Proteomics* **2014**, *14*, 1232–1238. [CrossRef] [PubMed]
10. Edwards, R.L.; Griffiths, P.; Bunch, J.; Cooper, H.J. Top-down proteomics and direct surface sampling of neonatal dried blood spots: Diagnosis of unknown hemoglobin variants. *J. Am. Soc. Mass Spectrom.* **2012**, *23*, 1921–1930. [CrossRef] [PubMed]
11. Edwards, R.L.; Creese, A.J.; Baumert, M.; Griffiths, P.; Bunch, J.; Cooper, H.J. Hemoglobin variant analysis via direct surface sampling of dried blood spots coupled with high-resolution mass spectrometry. *Anal. Chem.* **2011**, *15*, 2265–2270. [CrossRef] [PubMed]
12. Lobitz, S.; Telfer, P.; Cela, E.; Allaf, B.; Angastiniotis, M.; Backman Johansson, C.; Badens, C.; Bento, C.; Bouva, M.J.; Canatan, D.; et al. Newborn screening for sickle cell disease in Europe: Recommendations from a Pan-European consensus conference. *Br. J. Haematol.* **2018**. [CrossRef] [PubMed]

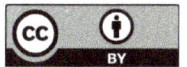

© 2019 by the authors. Licensee MDPI, Basel, Switzerland. This article is an open access article distributed under the terms and conditions of the Creative Commons Attribution (CC BY) license (http://creativecommons.org/licenses/by/4.0/).

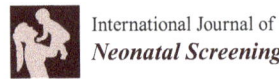

Article

Evaluation of Technical Issues in a Pilot Multicenter Newborn Screening Program for Sickle Cell Disease

Maddalena Martella [1,*], Giampietro Viola [1], Silvia Azzena [1], Sara Schiavon [1], Andrea Biondi [2], Giuseppe Basso [1], Paola Corti [2], Raffaella Colombatti [1], Nicoletta Masera [2] and Laura Sainati [1]

1. Dipartimento di Salute della Donna e del Bambino, Università di Padova, 35128 Padova, Italy; giampietro.viola.1@unipd.it (G.V.); azzena.silvia@yahoo.it (S.A.); schiavon_sara@libero.it (S.S.); giuseppe.basso@unipd.it (G.B.); rcolombatti@gmail.com (R.C.); laura.sainati@unipd.it (L.S.)
2. Dipartimento di Pediatria, Università di Milano-Bicocca-Fondazione MBBM, San Gerardo Hospital, 20900 Monza, Italy; abiondi.unimib@gmail.com (A.B.); p.corti@hsgerardo.org (P.C.); n.masera@hsgerardo.org (N.M.)
* Correspondence: maddalena.martella@unipd.it; Tel.: +39-49-8211451

Received: 30 October 2018; Accepted: 19 December 2018; Published: 21 December 2018

Abstract: A multicenter pilot program for universal newborn screening of Sickle cell disease (SCD) was conducted in two centres of Northern Italy (Padova and Monza). High Performance Liquid Chromatography (HPLC) was performed as the first test on samples collected on Guthrie cards and molecular analysis of the β-globin gene (*HBB*) was the confirmatory test performed on the HPLC-positive or indeterminate samples. 5466 samples of newborns were evaluated. Of these, 5439/5466 were submitted to HPLC analysis and the molecular analysis always confirmed in all the alteration detected in HPLC (62/5439 newborns); 4/5439 (0.07%) were SCD affected, 37/5439 (0.68%) were HbAS carriers and 21/5439 (0.40%) showed other hemoglobinopathies. Stored dried blood spots were adequate for HPLC and β-globin gene molecular analysis. Samples were suitable for analysis until sixteen months old. A cut-off of A_1 percentage, in order to avoid false negative or unnecessary confirmation tests, was identified. Our experience showed that several technical issues need to be addressed and resolved while developing a multicenter NBS program for SCD in a country where there is no national neonatal screening (NBS) program for SCD and NBS programs occur on a regional basis.

Keywords: sickle cell disease; high performance liquid chromatography (HPLC); β-globin gene

1. Introduction

Neonatal screening (NBS) for Sickle cell disease (SCD) is an effective tool for the early detection of affected individuals, to direct them at the clinical programs to prevent complications and finally to offer genetic counseling to a family and is therefore highly recommended as the first step of comprehensive care [1–7]. In detail, early identification of affected SCD patients through a NBS program allows the introduction of penicillin prophylaxis from two months of age and performing of an adequate vaccination schedule with the reduction of mortality from infection, prompt enrolment in comprehensive care programs with timely parent health education, Trans Cranial Doppler (TCD) screening and prevention of acute events [1,2].

In Italy a national NBS program is not available and NBS programs are organized on a regional basis [8]. Haemoglobinopathies are included in the regional NBS program of only 1 out of the 20 regions [9], but some pilot programs have been conducted in the past years [10–12].

Padova and Monza, two towns located in the North of Italy, in the Veneto and Lombardia Regions respectively, have a high percentage of an immigrant population and an average of more than 3500 births every year, with 25% of them from immigrant parents [13]. We developed a pilot multicenter, multiregional universal NBS program for SCD [14].

The methods used and recommended for the SCD neonatal screening by International Guidelines can be qualitative, as IsoElectric Focusing (IEF), and quantitative, as Capillary Electrophoresis (CE), High Performance Liquid Chromatography (HPLC) and recently the Tandem Mass Spectrometry (MS/MS) [15], but the abnormal chromatogram must always have a confirmatory test with the different methodologies. Our protocol is an innovative way for SCD screening with the combination of HPLC analysis and molecular analysis. This type of approach has been used in very few studies [16,17].

The purpose of this manuscript is to highlight some of the technical challenges that we had to face in the development of our pilot screening. The objectives of this study were: (i) to define the sensitivity of our methods in order to establish a cut-off percentage for normality in the presence of low levels of β-globin chains, (ii) to maintain high-quality results to ensure the accurate interpretation of the analysis for immediate initiation of supportive care for affected newborns, (iii) to check the stability of the sample over time to ensure reliable measurements, a very important issue in a multicenter setting, (iv) to verify the organization and feasibility of a multiregional screening program. Finally, the flow chart for newborn screening for SCD is shown in Figure 1.

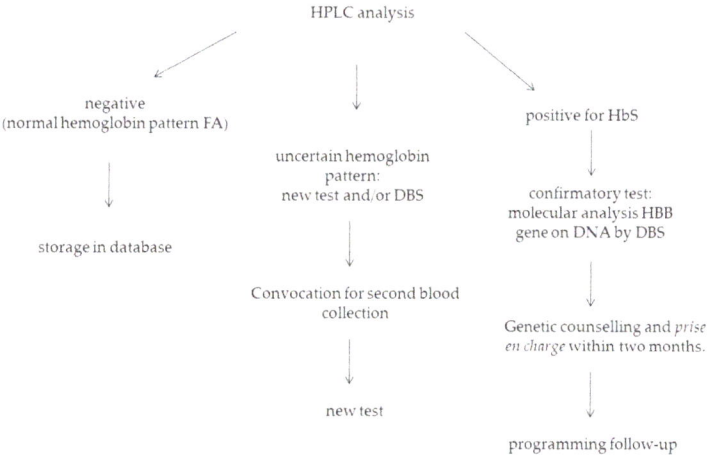

Figure 1. Flow chart for newborn screening for Sickle cell disease.

2. Materials and Methods

2.1. Study Design and Population

In Padova the NBS pilot program enrolled newborns from 2 May 2016 until 30 November 2017 while in Monza from 1 September 2016 until 31 August 2017. The screening was performed on all newborns from the 36th hour to the third day after birth. Blood collection was performed by pricking the heel of the newborn and collection on a Guthrie card (903 Whatman® in Padova and AHLSTROM® 226 in Monza) after informed consent from the parents was obtained.

Dried blood spots from Monza were sent to Padova through courier once a week and stored at room temperature and in a dark dry place in the NBS laboratory of Padova's Clinic of Pediatric Hematology-Oncology. The samples were analyzed after 7 days and the first test was performed with the VARIANT NBS Newborn Screening System (Bio-Rad Laboratories, Munich, Germany) and the confirmatory test, on the same sample, with molecular analysis of β-globin gene.

2.2. High Performance Liquid Chromatography (HPLC)

All specimens were first examined by High Performance Liquid Chromatography (HPLC) performed on a VARIANT NBS Newborn Screening System (Bio-Rad Laboratories) following the manufacturer's recommendations, within 7 days after blood spots had been taken. All chromatograms were automatically analyzed and visually inspected for absent Hemoglobin A and variant hemoglobins. The columns and all reagents such as buffers, primers, and hemoglobin standards were purchased from the manufacturer. Two or three disks (diameter of 3.2 mm) were punched out of the dried blood spot (DBS) and placed in a well of 96-well plate round bottom. In each well 280μL of distilled water was added and mixed with the pipette several times at room temperature. Two mixtures of hemoglobin standards FAES and FADC, respectively were analyzed in duplicate even if the run included more plates.

HPLC uses an ion exchange column with gradient elution. The presence of different hemoglobins is revealed through a UV-VIS detector settled at 415 nm. The time that passes from the injection of the sample to the output of the peak of hemoglobin type, is known as the retention time of that particular hemoglobin and represents a reproducible value for that column, at that gradient elution and at that temperature. For the different hemoglobins we have different retention times and characteristic chromatographic profiles, with the exception of HbE and HbA_2 that elute in the same peak, therefore making them indistinguishable from each other.

In addition, it is possible to quantify in a relative way the percentage of the different hemoglobins; the HPLC analysis helps to identify the differences between carrier individuals (HbS/HbA) and homozygous affected individuals (HbS/HbS) and also to differentiate heterozygous compounds such as HbS/HbC.

Moreover, the sensibility of the protocol has been verified with experiments of dilution on the SCD sample (HbSS) until 1:10.

2.3. Molecular Analysis of the β-globin Gene

Molecular analysis of the β-globin gene (*HBB*; MIM # 603903; NM_000518) represented the confirmatory test and was performed on all the following samples: those with an altered hemoglobin profile at HPLC, due to the presence of HbS or another hemoglobin variant; the specimens with HbA<5% or with HbA>30%, excluded transfusion anamnesis, were sent for molecular study. The samples with a red blood cell transfusion and HbA>30% were submitted for HPLC analysis three months later.

Genomic DNA, extracted using the Qiagen kit (QIAamp®DNA Mini and Blood), from blood spots allowed to air dry, were amplified by chain reaction of polymerase (PCR) at the exon level and at the intron-exon junctions with the primers below reported: *HBB1* Fw5'-AAAAGTCAGGGCAGAGCCAT-3', *HBB1* Rw5'-CCCAGTTTCTATTGGTCTCCTTAA-3', *HBB2* Fw5'-GGGTTTCTGATAGGCACTGACTC-3', *HBB2* Rw5'-AAAAGAAGGGGAAAGAAAACATCA-3', *HBB3* Fw5'-TAGCAGCTACAATCCAGCTACCA-3', *HBB3* Rw5'-GGACTTAGGGAACAAAGGACCT-3'.

Alterations of the coding sequence were analyzed and characterized by sequencing of the hemoglobin β chain coding *HBB* gene using an ABI Prism® 310 Genetic Analyzer Applied Biosystems. Sanger sequencing is the most comprehensive method of mutation detection and determines the exact sequence spanning the area of the primers used.

2.4. Management of Results

HPLC negative samples for abnormal hemoglobins didn't require further analysis. While, HPLC positive samples for abnormal chains underwent a confirmatory test with molecular analysis of the β-globin gene on the same sample collected at the nursery. Families with SCD children were called for a visit in the clinic within two months, while parents of HbS carriers were called for a visit and counselling within six months. Carriers of other hemoglobin variants received a letter, informing them of the results.

3. Results

In this study, 5466 samples of newborns from both birth centers were enrolled. Of these, 5439/5466 (2821/2826 of Padova, 99.8% and 2618/2640 of Monza 99.1%) were submitted for HPLC analysis. None of the samples collected were excluded from the analysis. Each sample was analyzed within 7 days after the blood had been spotted on the paper.

The results are summarized in Table 1. Molecular analysis always confirmed the abnormality detected in HPLC in 62/5466 newborns; other hemoglobin variants were also detected (HbC, HbD, HbE) in 0.5% of the cases in Monza and in 0.21% of those in Padova.

Table 1. Hemoglobin patterns observed in the pilot newborn screening.

Hb Pattern (HPLC)	HBB Genotype	Newborns (n.)
FAS	HBB: c.20A>T/wt	37 (0.68%)
FS	HBB: c.20A>T/c.20A>T	3 (0.055%)
FSC	HBB: c.20A>T/c.19A>T	1 (0.02%)
FAC	HBB: c.19A>T/wt	9 (0.16%)
FAD	HBB: c.364G>C/wt	8 (0.15%)
FAE	HBB: c.79C>T/wt	4 (0.07%)
	Total	62 (1.14%)

n. = number of newborns.

28 samples (0.86%) of preterm infants, showed a value of HbA<5% at HPLC. Molecular analysis confirmed that 26/28 had genotype HbAA, while 2 samples with HbA values of 2.2% and 3.8%, respectively, had a genotype HbAD and a FAST value >10% (potential HbBart) and had been reported to the referring center. In an attempt to determine normal values for HbA and total HbF, the peak percentages of samples with a normal hemoglobin pattern were plotted against the gestational week. The results (see Figure 2) showed a correct Gaussian distribution for the HbA and HbF with a mean of 16.6% and 77.1% respectively as expected for at term newborns.

All dried blood spot cards collected and the storage methods turned out adequate both for HPLC analysis and β globin gene molecular analysis.

The experiments of dilution on the SCD sample (HbSS) detected low levels of HbS until 1:10.

In our experience we verified storage conditions and the reliability of the DBS a few months later [16] to understand if it was possible to identify the different hemoglobins according to our standard settings of the instrument. We repeated the HPLC analysis of different DBS series stored for sixteen months. In each series, the values of HbA peak area percentage identified in HPLC analysis, although reduced, allowed for the detection of the hemoglobin peaks; retention time was not modified by the samples aging: the HbA value was never <7% and never <800,000 µV*s, in terms of area under the curve (AUC) according to manufacturer instructions. HbS, when present was easily identified by HPLC analysis and similarly to HbA it was not influenced by sample aging [18]. The reduction of the HbA percentage should be attributed to physiological degradation of HbA and to the presence of cellulose particles removed from the Guthrie card together with the blood. In this study, the DBS up to sixteen months old provided satisfactory results (see Figure 3). The quality and the efficiency of the analysis was not affected by different types of Guthrie cards and the two different types of Guthrie cards gave the same performance.

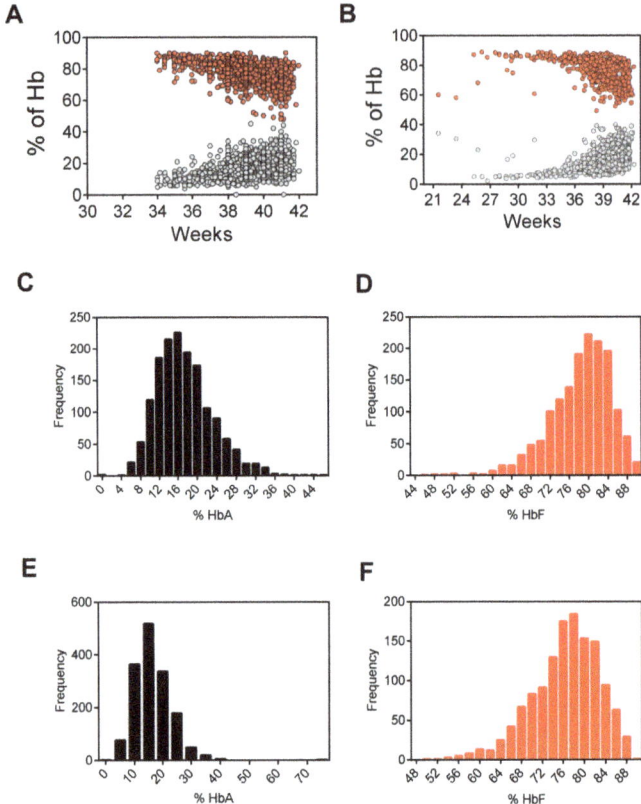

Figure 2. Percentages of HbF (red circles) and HbA (gray circles) according to the gestational age (weeks from conception to blood withdrawal) found in the cohort of Padova (**A**) and Monza (**B**). Distribution frequency of HbA and HbF in the cohort of Padova (**C,D**) and Monza (**E,F**).

Furthermore, we have noted in our experience that the needle restrains randomly, probably by electrostatic reasons, some blood spots that could cause not only the obstruction of the needle, but also the contamination of other wells. Thus, we recommend that the run must be always monitored and if necessary the run should be interrupted. At the end of every analysis session the instrument must be carefully cleaned.

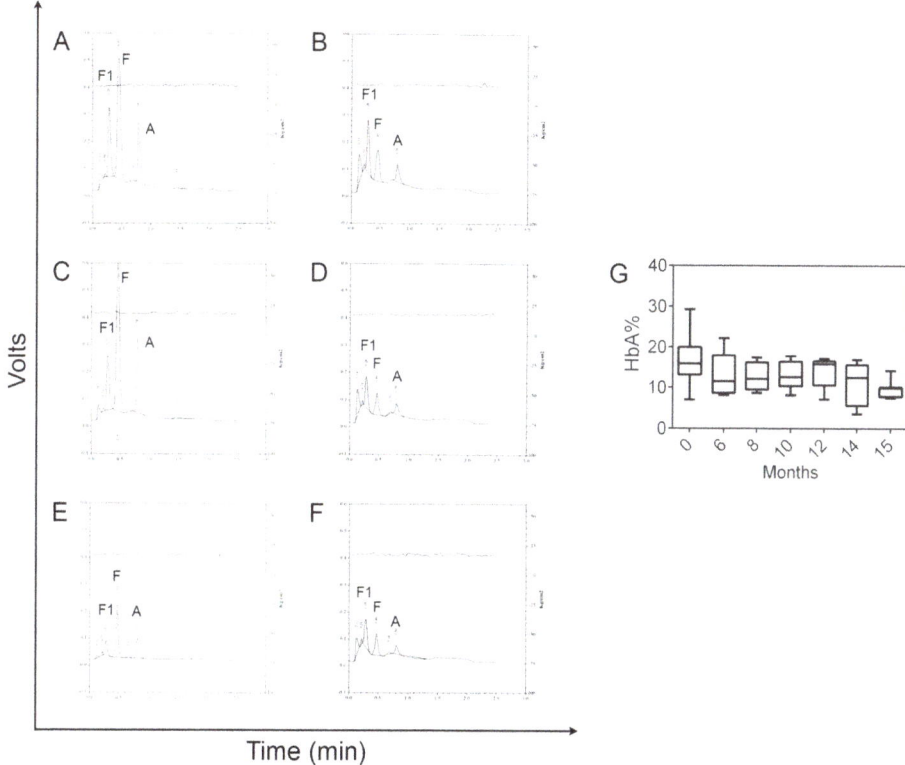

Figure 3. Representative chromatograms of a dried blood spot analyzed within 7 days from blood withdrawal (**A**,**C**,**E**) and after four (**B**), eight (**D**) and sixteen months (**F**). Percentages of HbA analyzed after different months from the blood withdrawal (**G**). At least five samples for group were analyzed.

4. Discussion

Our study represents the first multicenter pilot project of universal NBS for SCD in two different regions of Northern Italy.

The methods of investigation were adequate and highly specific, the confirmatory test always confirmed the abnormal hemoglobinopathies detected in HPLC. The two different types of Guthrie cards gave the same performances. The quality, the storage of the sample and the volume of the collected blood are very important factors that may affect the results in particular the retention time in HPLC of the different hemoglobins [19]. Our setting proved to be effective.

Moreover, in our experience we noted that it is very important for the setting of the 96-well plate for HPLC analysis to ensure the acquisition of the total area >800,000 µV*s, as recommended by the manufacture: The number of the spots, the volume of the water for Hb elution, mixed with the pipette several times at room temperature. The 96-well plate can be store at room temperature. This protocol ensures a homogeneous solution to detect the different hemoglobins. The sensitivity of the system can be considered optimal for all different hemoglobins in agreement with the hemoglobin standards FAES and FADC provided by the manufacturer. It is worthwhile to note that our data showed a normal distribution both for HbA and HbF in well agreement to that reported by Bouva et al. [20].

Finally, the sensibility of the protocol verified with experiments of dilution on the SCD sample (HbSS) until 1:10 guaranteed the possibility of detecting low levels of HbS.

Newborns born prematurely may yield misleading results. Premature infants may have very low levels of A_1 hemoglobin at birth; in the absence of a significant amount of A_1, β chains mutations can be undetectable. The cut-off of HbA<5% is efficient also for preterm newborns. The percentages of HbA and HbF were in agreement with previous reports [21,22], which found a great variability according to the maternal ethnic origin and the gestational age.

The VARIANT NBS Newborn Screening System for our experience has critical issues: the spots can remain attached to the needle causing obstruction or even the random fall of the spot. Therefore, caution is necessary and it is better to check the run and to wash frequently the needle and the instrument.

5. Conclusions

Our data demonstrate the feasibility of a multicentric SCD screening and indicate the robustness and reliability of the screening system. The data obtained from HPLC analysis were in excellent agreement with the large amount of data present in the literature. The sensitivity of the system can be considered optimal in conjunction with the molecular analysis of the β globin gene. A scaling up of the project to other areas of the two regions is now planned.

Author Contributions: Conceptualization, data curation, original draft preparation M.M. and G.V.; investigation, S.A. and S.S.; resources, G.B. and A.B.; project administration, N.M. and P.C.; L.S. and R.C. supervision, project administration and writing—review and editing.

Funding: The research was supported through a grant from Team for Children Onlus and one from the Fondazione MBBM (Monza e Brianza per il Bambino e la sua Mamma).

Conflicts of Interest: The authors declare no conflicts of interest.

References

1. Ware, R.E.; de Montalembert, M.; Tshilolo, L.; Abboud, M.R. Sickle cell disease. *Lancet* **2017**, *390*, 311–323. [CrossRef]
2. Piel, F.B.; Steinberg, M.H.; Rees, D.C. Sickle Cell Disease. *N. Engl. J. Med.* **2017**, *376*, 1561–1573. [CrossRef] [PubMed]
3. National Health System (NHS). Sicke Cell Disease in Childhood. Standard and Guidelines for clinical Care. 2nd Edition 2010. Available online: https://assets.publishing.service.gov.uk/government/uploads/system/uploads/attachment_data/file/408961/1332-SC-Clinical-Standards-WEB.pdf (accessed on 20 December 2018).
4. De Montalembert, M.; Ferster, A.; Colombatti, R.; Rees, D.C.; Gulbis, B. European Network for Rare and Congenital Anemias. ENERCA clinical recommendations for disease management and prevention of complications of sickle cell disease in children. *Am J. Hematol.* **2011**, *86*, 72–75. [CrossRef] [PubMed]
5. Colombatti, R.; Perrotta, S.; Samperi, P.; Casale, M.; Masera, N.; Palazzi, G.; Sainati, L.; Russo, G.; Italian Association of Pediatric Hematology-Oncology (AIEOP) Sickle Cell Disease Working Group. Organizing national responses for rare blood disorders: The Italian experience with sickle cell disease in childhood. *Orphanet J. Rare Dis.* **2013**, *8*, 169. [CrossRef] [PubMed]
6. De Franceschi, L.R.G.; Sainati, L.; Venturelli, D. SITE-AIEOP Recommendations for Sickle Cell Disease Neonatal Screening. Collana Scientifica Site n°5. Available online: http://www.site-italia.org/collana_scientifica.php (accessed on 20 December 2018).
7. Lobitz, S.; Telfer, P.; Cela, E.; Allaf, B.; Angastiniotis, M.; Backman, J.C.; Badens, C.; Bento, C.; Bouva, M.J.; Canatan, D.; et al. Newborn screening for sickle cell disease in Europe: Recommendations from a Pan-European Consensus Conference. *Br. J. Haematol.* **2018**, *183*, 648–660. [CrossRef] [PubMed]
8. Available online: http://www.aismme.org (accessed on 20 December 2018).
9. De Zen, L.; Dall'Amico, R.; Sainati, L.; Colombatti, R.; Testa, E.R.; Catapano, R.; Zanolli, F. Screening neonatale per le emoglobinopatie su Dried Blood Spot. In Proceedings of the XXXVI Congresso Nazionale Associazione Italiana Ematologia Oncologia Pediatrica (AIEOP), Pisa, Italy, 6–8 June 2010.
10. Rolla, R.; Castagno, M.; Zaffaroni, M.; Grigollo, B.; Colombo, S.; Piccotti, S.; Dellora, C.; Bona, G.; Bellomo, G. Neonatal screening for sickle cell disease and other hemoglobinopathies in "the changing Europe". *Clin. Lab.* **2014**, *60*, 2089–2093. [CrossRef] [PubMed]
11. Venturelli, D.; Lodi, M.; Palazzi, G.; Bergonzini, G.; Doretto, G.; Zini, A.; Monica, C.; Cano, M.C.; Ilaria, M.; Montagnani, G.; et al. Sickle cell disease in areas of immigration of high-risk populations: A low cost and reproducible method of screening in northern Italy. *Blood Transfus.* **2014**, *12*, 346–351. [PubMed]

12. Ballardini, E.; Tarocco, A.; Marsella, M.; Bernardoni, R.; Carandina, G.; Melandri, C.; Guerra, G.; Patella, A.; Zucchelli, M.; Ferlini, A.; et al. Universal neonatal screening for sickle cell disease and other haemoglobinopathies in Ferrara, Italy. *Blood Transfus.* **2013**, *11*, 245–249. [PubMed]
13. RapportoAnnuale ISTAT. 2017. Available online: https://www.istat.it/it/files//2017/05/RapportoAnnuale2017.pdf (accessed on 20 December 2018).
14. Martella, M.; Cattaneo, L.; Viola, G.; Azzena, S.; Cappellari, A.; Baraldi, E.; Zorloni, C.; Masera, N.; Biondi, A.; Basso, G.; et al. Universal Newborn Screening for Sickle Cell Disease: Preliminary Results of the First Year of a Multicentric Italian Project. In Proceedings of the 22nd Annual Congress of the European Hematology Association, Madrid, Spain, 22–25 June 2017.
15. Lobitz, S.; Klein, J.; Brose, A.; Blankenstein, O.; Frömmel, C. Newborn screening by tandem mass spectrometry confirms the high prevalence of sickle cell disease among German newborns. *Ann. Hematol.* **2017**, *23*, 1–6. [CrossRef] [PubMed]
16. Detemmerman, L.; Olivier, S.; Bours, V.; Boemer, F. Innovative PCR without DNA extraction for African sickle cell disease diagnosis. *Hematology* **2017**, *23*, 181–186. [CrossRef] [PubMed]
17. Kunz, J.B.; Awad, S.; Happich, M.; Muckenthaler, L.; Lindner, M.; Gramer, G.; Okun, J.G.; Hoffmann, G.F.; Bruckner, T.; Muckenthaler, M.U.; et al. Significant prevalence of sickle cell disease in Southwest Germany: Results from a birth cohort study indicate the necessity for newborn screening. *Ann. Hematol.* **2016**, *95*, 397–402. [CrossRef] [PubMed]
18. Martella, M.; Viola, G. Università di Padova, Padova, Italy. Chromatograms derived from HPLC analysis. Unpublish work, 2018.
19. Frömmel, C.; Brose, A.; Klein, J.; Blankenstein, O.; Lobitz, S. Newborn Screening for Sickle Cell Disease: Technical and Legal Aspects of a German Pilot Study with 38,220 Participants. *BioMed Res. Int.* **2014**, *2014*, 695828. [CrossRef] [PubMed]
20. Bouva, M.J.; Mohrmann, K.; Brinkman, H.B.J.M.; Kemper-Proper, E.A.; Elvers, B.; Loeber, J.G.; Verheul, F.E.A.M.; Giordano, P.C. Implementing neonatal screening for haemoglobinopathies in the Netherlands. *J. Med. Screen.* **2010**, *17*, 58–65. [CrossRef] [PubMed]
21. CorteÂs-Castell, E.; PalazoÂn-Bru, A.; Pla, C.; Goicoechea, M.; Rizo-Baeza, M.M.; Juste, M.; Gil-Guillen, V.F. Impact of prematurity and immigration on neonatal screening for sickle cell disease. *PLoS ONE* **2017**, *12*, e0171604. [CrossRef] [PubMed]
22. Allaf, B.; Patin, F.; Elion, J.; Couque, N. New approach to accurate interpretation of sickle cell disease newborn screening by applying multiple of median cutoffs and ratios. *Pediatr. Blood Cancer* **2018**, *65*, e27230. [CrossRef] [PubMed]

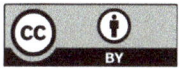

© 2018 by the authors. Licensee MDPI, Basel, Switzerland. This article is an open access article distributed under the terms and conditions of the Creative Commons Attribution (CC BY) license (http://creativecommons.org/licenses/by/4.0/).

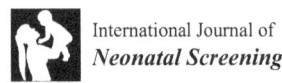

Review

Newborn Screening for Sickle Cell Disease in Europe

Yvonne Daniel [1,†,*], Jacques Elion [2,†], Bichr Allaf [3], Catherine Badens [4], Marelle J. Bouva [5], Ian Brincat [6], Elena Cela [7], Cathy Coppinger [1], Mariane de Montalembert [8], Béatrice Gulbis [9], Joan Henthorn [1], Olivier Ketelslegers [10], Corrina McMahon [11], Allison Streetly [12,13], Raffaella Colombatti [14,†] and Stephan Lobitz [15,†]

1. Public Health England, NHS Sickle Cell and Thalassemia Screening Programme, London SE16LH, UK; Cathy.Coppinger@phe.gov.uk (C.C.); joan.henthorn@gmail.com (J.H.)
2. Laboratoire d'Excellence GR-Ex, UMR_S1134, Inserm, Université Paris Diderot, Sorbonne Paris Cité, Institut National de la Transfusion Sanguine, 75015 Paris, France; jacques.elion@inserm.fr
3. NBS Laboratory for Haemoglobinopathies, Hôpital Universitaire Robert-Debré, 75019 Paris, France; bichr.allaf@aphp.fr
4. Département de génétique médicale, Aix-Marseille Université, Hôpital de la Timone, 13385 Marseille, France; catherine.badens@ap-hm.fr
5. National Institute for Public Health and the Environment, Centre for Health Protection, 3720 Bilthoven, The Netherlands; marelle.bouva@rivm.nl
6. Pediatric Medicine Laboratory, Department of Pathology, Mater Dei Hospital, Triq Tal-Qroqq, MSD2090 Msida, Malta; ian.brincat@gov.mt
7. Department of Pediatric Oncology/Hematology, Hospital Universitario General Gregorio Marañón, Facultad de Medicina, Universidad Complutense Madrid, 28007 Madrid, Spain; elena.cela@salud.madrid.org
8. Department of Pediatrics, Reference Center for Sickle Cell Disease, AP-HP Hôpital Universitaire Necker-Enfants Malades, 75743 Paris, France; mariane.demontal@aphp.fr
9. Department of Clinical Chemistry, Cliniques Universitaires de Bruxelles, Hôpital Erasme—ULB, 1070 Bruxelles, Belgium; beatrice.gulbis@erasme.ulb.ac.be
10. Laboratoire—Biologie Clinique, Centre Hospitalier Régional de la Citadelle, 4000 Liège, Belgium; Olivier.ketelslegers@chrcitadelle.be
11. Our Lady's Children's Hospital, Crumlin, D12V004 Dublin, Ireland; corrina.mcmahon@olchc.ie
12. School of Population Health and Environmental Sciences, Faculty of Life Sciences & Medicine, King's College London, London WC2R2LS, UK; allison.streetly@phe.gov.uk
13. Division of Healthcare Public Health, Health Protection and Medical Directorate, Public Health England, London SE18UG, UK
14. Department of Child and Maternal Health, Clinic of Pediatric Hematology/Oncology, Azienda Ospedaliera-Università di Padova, 35129 Padova, Italy; rcolombatti@gmail.com
15. Department of Pediatric Oncology/Hematology, Kinderkrankenhaus Amsterdamer Straße, 50735 Cologne, Germany; lobitzs@kliniken-koeln.de
* Correspondence: yvonne.a.daniel@kcl.ac.uk
† These authors contributed equally to the manuscript.

Received: 30 December 2018; Accepted: 6 February 2019; Published: 12 February 2019

Abstract: The history of newborn screening (NBS) for sickle cell disease (SCD) in Europe goes back almost 40 years. However, most European countries have not established it to date. The European screening map is surprisingly heterogenous. The first countries to introduce sickle cell screening on a national scale were France and England. The French West Indies started to screen their newborns for SCD as early as 1983/84. To this day, all countries of the United Kingdom of Great Britain and Northern Ireland have added SCD as a target disease to their NBS programs. The Netherlands, Spain and Malta also have national programs. Belgium screens regionally in the Brussels and Liège regions, Ireland has been running a pilot for many years that has become quasi-official. However, the Belgian and Irish programs are not publicly funded. Italy and Germany have completed several pilot studies but are still in the preparatory phase of national NBS programs for SCD, although both countries have well-established concepts for metabolic and endocrine disorders. This article will give a brief overview of the situation in Europe and put a focus on the programs of the two pioneers of the continent, England and France.

Keywords: screening; sickle cell disease; newborn

---

1. England

1.1. Historical Background

Newborn screening (NBS) for sickle cell disease (SCD) was implemented in England between 2002 and 2005. Migration to the United Kingdom (UK) after 1945 had led to an increase in the population at risk from SCD, whilst the 1972 USA National Sickle Cell Anemia Control Act [1] had resulted in increased recognition and politicization of the disorder. The 1986 randomized trial of penicillin in SCD children aged less than 5 by Gaston et al. [2] demonstrated improved outcomes and provided a clear justification for NBS for SCD. Pockets of NBS had been implemented locally in some high prevalence areas in the 1970s but these were not systematic and resulted in inequitable policies throughout the country. These factors led to a major review by a Health Technology Assessment [3] working party which formed the basis for subsequent policy decisions. Political commitment was achieved via the National Health Service (NHS) plan in 2000 [4] and this led to the formation of a small team to plan and drive implementation of a linked newborn and antenatal screening program.

At this time, despite political commitment there were no policies and no financial resources had been allocated. Funding was only able to be sourced once an implementation plan had been developed. The working group had to resolve the controversy and sensitivities associated with implementing a genetic test in a minority group along with resistance from some who questioned the value of the program. There was also conflict between the desires of stakeholders and what could realistically be achieved. Initially overseas practices were reviewed, and a survey of local practices was carried out to inform decisions. A steering group was established in 2001, comprised of key health professionals, users and representatives from patient groups to endorse the policy decisions put forward by the expert working sub groups. Sub groups were developed to work on specific issues such as training, laboratory practices, education and information for users and professionals. The UK National Screening Committee makes recommendations to ministers about all decisions regarding screening policy in the UK and in 2002 approval was given for universal screening of SCD in children. The techniques in use also detected other hemoglobinopathies including beta thalassemia disease (defined clinically as transfusion dependent beta thalassemia or non-transfusion dependent beta thalassemia or HbE/beta thalassemia) thus it was also agreed that these cases along with all other hemoglobin variants detected would be reported. Policy was subsequently updated following review in 2011 such that the only other haemoglobins now reported are beta thalassemia disease, hemoglobins S, C, D, E and O^{Arab}, along with any variant co-inherited with Hb S. The four countries which form the UK operate semi-autonomously and screening in Scotland, Northern Ireland and Wales was adopted later. Scotland and Northern Ireland broadly follow the English policy whilst Wales implemented screening much later and has its own strategy [5].

1.2. Implementation

Along with stakeholder engagement, initial work was related to the development of policies for implementation. These covered areas such as sample type, technology to be used, testing protocols, reporting, delivery of results and referral into care. It was agreed that the blood spot sample already collected for metabolic screening would be used and that the program would be incorporated into the newborn blood spot screening pathway. Following reorganization there were 13 laboratories performing NBS in England, and thus implementation required policies which ensured consistency as well as a significant training investment. A two-stage testing protocol was implemented to increase the robustness of data with only high-performance liquid chromatography (HPLC) and iso-electric focusing (IEF) recognized as acceptable techniques (https://www.gov.uk/government/publications/sickle-cell-and-thalassemia-screening-handbook-for-laboratories). Counselling was aligned with genetics and different models were developed to fit with local prevalence of the conditions, resources and practices. Areas with high incidence had dedicated counsellors. Clinical policies and standards were developed, and these were subsequently published (https://www.gov.uk/government/publications/sickle-cell-disease-in-children-standards-for-clinical-care). Some funds were provided towards the development of initiatives such as transcranial Doppler scanning. Standards and the key performance indicators to measure performance against these standards were introduced (https://www.gov.uk/government/publications/standards-for-sickle-cell-and-thalassaemia-screening). The standards have evolved over time and are now reviewed annually to ensure they remain fit for purpose. A communication strategy is an important aspect to ensure engagement in the process. Educational materials such as booklets and leaflets for professionals, parents and the public (available in different languages) were developed. More recently blogs and other online resources have been used. Information and educational resources were developed for professionals and a variety of education and training for NHS screening staff is available (https://www.gov.uk/guidance/sickle-cell-and-thalassaemia-screening-education-and-training#haemoglobinopathies-sct-screening-programme-update).

Annual data collection and reporting has been developed and the information is used to inform decisions and to monitor trends, performance and the effect of changes in practice. Quality assurance of the whole pathway via peer review and inspection has been an important factor in ensuring consistency and maintaining standards. The ongoing evaluation present since the program's inception has led to the development of initiatives such as a failsafe to ensure samples are received on all babies and provision for the testing of babies who have been transfused. An initiative to measure outcomes from early detection of SCD in England was commenced in 2010 and has subsequently reported [6].

1.3. Results

More than 8 million babies have now been screened in the England; 3686 screen positive babies were identified between 2005 and 31 March 2017 [6], a summary of results is shown in Table 1.

Table 1. Screen positive babies between 2005 and 31 March 2017.

Screening Result	Number	Percentage
FS	2580	70.0%
FSC	927	25.1%
FS + other hemoglobin variant *	179	4.9%

* Refers to Hb D, E, O^{Arab} and any other rare variants detected.

The recently published newborn outcomes project which assessed timeliness of entry into care and treatment, antenatal screening history, and mortality reported on 1313 screen positive infants [6]. The paper concludes that the screening program accurately identifies babies with SCD, enrolment into care is timely but does not meet program standards, and despite mortality being low deaths still occur from invasive pneumococcal disease with adherence to antibiotics remaining important.

1.4. Summary

The long road from the first pockets of screening to full implementation of universal NBS for SCD in the whole of the UK took almost 30 years. Initially implementation was in England followed by Scotland, Northern Ireland and eventually Wales in 2014. Implementation was driven by increasing immigration and public pressure for inclusion in health care strategy. Testing for SCD is now firmly embedded in newborn blood spot screening which is assessed as a complete pathway rather than individual components. Additionally as part of linked antenatal and newborn screening, the program acts as a quality measure for antenatal screening with any apparent discrepancies being investigated. A key element in the success of the program has been the input of the small team who have driven the process, and ensured and maintained stakeholder engagement and development and implementation of policies. Ongoing evaluation and assessment is an essential aspect to ensure the program is fit for purpose. The program has proven itself to be adaptable, for example by adopting new technologies such as mass spectrometry testing [7,8]. The use of the new technology to withhold detection of carrier conditions has led to differing strategies in the UK. Within England, consistency has been maintained despite some adoption of this technique. Balancing all stakeholder expectations and requirements continues to be a challenge in the program.

The newborn outcomes project has shown that the program accurately identifies babies with SCD but there are some issues including acceptance of penicillin and delays between babies' positive screening results and enrolment into care and mortality associated with invasive pneumococcal disease. A detailed review into all aspects of the process and stakeholder requirements (a discovery process), identified a lack of a centralized view of the baby's progress along the pathway, lack of feedback to data providers, and duplication of data entry. A new improved system has been developed which will:

1. Automate the process of referring screen-positive babies into treatment centres and record their health outcomes;
2. Help ensure affected babies are treated as early as possible;
3. Provide oversight of the progress along the pathway to prevent babies getting 'lost' in the system;
4. Improve the process of collecting and sharing data;
5. Remove the need for clinicians to enter the same data twice;
6. Integrate with the National Hemoglobinopathy Register and National Congenital Anomalies and Rare Disorders Registration Service.

Beta thalassemia continues to be reported when found in NBS for SCD, and this has been due to lack of available evidence on the efficacy of detection and the clinical justification for early detection. There is now improved evidence on the sensitivity and specificity of the test [9,10]. However published clinical evidence remains scarce.

In conclusion, over 10 years' experience in England has shown this to be a robust program, which benefits from technical expertise along with strong stakeholder engagement. A key aspect of the program's success has been the development of clinical care pathways to ensure screen positive babies receive appropriate care in a timely manner.

2. France

2.1. Historical Background and Implementation

The first pilot study on NBS for SCD in France was conducted on the Caribbean island of Guadeloupe in 1983 and led to a universal screening program in Guadeloupe within one year [11]. The program was rapidly extended to Martinique, and in 1986 the first pilot studies in Metropolitan France (Paris and Marseille) were started.

In 1995, SCD became an additional target disease of the national NBS program in France (together with phenylketonuria, congenital hypothyroidism, congenital adrenal hyperplasia and cystic fibrosis). However, although the French NBS is universal in nature, screening for SCD in Metropolitan France is targeted at couples at risk to date, while in French overseas territories SCD screening is universal [12].

NBS for SCD is centralized in France and performed in five reference laboratories. Three of these are located in Metropolitan France (Paris, Marseille, Lille) and two are run on the Caribbean islands of Guadeloupe and Martinique. Since the year 2000, all French maternity clinics (public and private) are covered by the program which receives funding from the French social security system.

2.2. Methods

NBS for SCD in France is done in a two-tier strategy from heel prick dried blood spots. Initially, IEF was the method of choice. Today, the first-tier methods are HPLC, capillary electrophoresis (CE) and very recently MALDI-TOF mass spectrometry found its way into NBS in one laboratory. Second-tier testing is done with an established method different from the first one (e.g., first-tier: HPLC; second-tier: CE). The United Kingdom National External Quality Assessment Service (UK NEQAS) provides the external quality control assessment for the French NBS program. Absolute numbers of new cases, incidence, coverage and genotypes are collected and published annually globally and for each of the French regions (http://www.afdphe.org/sites/default/files/bilan_afdphe_2016.pdf). Screening results consistent with SCD are communicated to the families by a trained pediatrician of the national care program. Parents of carriers are informed by mail and offered information by a physician or a genetic counsellor. Testing of the father is recommended to identify couples at risk of having a significant disorder of hemoglobin. In this latter context, genetic counselling including extended information on SCD is provided and the opportunities of having prenatal or preimplantation genetic diagnosis are mentioned. A psychologist will participate in the process whenever necessary.

2.3. Results

Between the beginning of the national program in 1995 and 2016, 5.4 million newborns have been screened and 7,644 of tested newborns were diagnosed with SCD. A summary of results is shown in Table 2.

Table 2. Screen positive babies between 1995 and 2016.

Screening Result	Number	Percentage
FS	6015	78.7%
FSC	1600	20.9%
FS + other hemoglobin variant *	29	0.4%

* Refers to Hb D, E, O^{Arab} and any other rare variants detected.

In 2016, 431 cases of SCD were identified by NBS which corresponded with a birth prevalence of 1 in 1836, i.e., the highest among all target diseases tested in the French national NBS program. 356 of these 431 cases were diagnosed in Metropolitan France, and 218 of the 356 cases in Metropolitan France were diagnosed in the Ile de France, i.e., in the Parisian area. This translated into a birth prevalence of 1 in 824 in the Ile de France. In the French Overseas, 75 babies were affected by SCD. This was a mean birth prevalence of 1 in 525, varying from 1 in 1968 on the Island of Réunion and 1 in 206 in French Guiana (http://www.afdphe.org/sites/default/files/bilan_afdphe_2016.pdf).

The birth coverage by universal NBS in the French Overseas is over 98%. In the targeted program of Metropolitan France, a mean of 38.9% of all newborns was screened in 2016 (minimum: 9.1% in the Brittany region; maximum: 73.6% in the Ile de France). Only 277 parents (0.035%) refused to participate to the French NBS program in 2016. Between 2006 and 2016, there was a significant increase of couples at risk that led to a subsequent increase of the newborns screened in the targeted program in Metropolitan France from 27 to 38.9% (see above). In the same period, the prevalence of affected newborns rose by 24%.

The targeted SCD NBS in Metropolitan France is probably more cost-effective than a universal approach. The present cost per test is EUR 3.06. This equals to total costs of EUR 1.02 million per year for the whole program or EUR 2,359 per newborn identified. However, there are several drawbacks: most importantly, about 2% of affected newborns are missed, because they are not screened for various reasons [13]. Hence, patients' associations and most of the concerned medical health care professionals advocate a universal screening approach. Beyond missed cases, arguments in favor of universal screening include putative discrimination and inequality to the access to care. Still, in its December

2013 orientation report the *Haute Autorité de Santé* concluded that there is currently no evidence to justify universal NBS for SCD in Metropolitan France.

2.4. Follow-Up and Organization of Care

The first French Sickle Cell Disease Comprehensive Care Center was established in Guadeloupe in 1990 [11]. In 2005, a pioneering national program on rare diseases was started in France. Its objectives include the definition of pathways to access to care, the prevention of diagnostic wavering, the establishment of reference centers, the organization of specialized training for health care professionals, the development of information platforms for patients, relatives, health care professionals and the community, and the promotion of research.

During the first phase of this program (2005–2008), two accredited reference centers for SCD (Ile de France and French Antilles), one reference center for thalassemia (Marseille) and a network of reference laboratories were founded. The mission of these institutions was to establish clear healthcare channels for the patients through the formation of a national network of qualified centers. In 2005, national treatment guidelines for SCD were published online.

In the second phase of the national program for rare diseases (2011–2014), 13 constitutive reference centers and 46 competence centers in addition to the coordination reference centers were established to ensure a dense and comprehensive coverage of the whole French national territory.

A national registry for thalassemias has been established that included 692 patients (beta thalassemia: 612; alpha thalassemia: 80) in 2016, but a national registry for SCD is only now being established. (Definitions: beta thalassemia = transfusion dependent beta thalassemia or non-transfusion dependent beta thalassemia or HbE/beta thalassemia; alpha thalassemia = alpha thalassemia hydrops fetalis syndrome, HbH disease and HbH-Constant Spring disease.)

The whole network was certified in 2017 for five years. The program is evaluated regularly for its efficiency by health authorities and through published studies [14,15] and the next turn of certification is to occur in 2022.

In addition, local networks have been established at the initiative of some dedicated physicians, like RoFSED (*Réseau Francilien de Soin des Enfants Drépanocytaires*) in the Parisian area, and supported by public funds to connect the national health care system with proximity stakeholders, e.g., general practitioners, local health care and social professionals and school personnel. They are essential actors in terms of therapeutic education of the patients and parents and information of the general public (e.g., brochures, educational sessions and tools, games, films etc.; for examples, please see: http://www.rofsed.fr).

3. The Netherlands

The Netherlands has had a national NBS since 1974. Participation is voluntary, but virtually all of the newborns (approximately 175,000 annually) are tested. Since 2015 also newborns from the Dutch Caribbean, Bonaire, St Eustatius and Saba (200–250 children), are screened. For this, the specimens are sent to one of the five designated NBS laboratories in The Netherlands. Specimens are heel prick dried blood spots that are currently examined for 19 conditions. 16 of which are endocrine and metabolic disorders. The other three are blood disorders. NBS for SCD was introduced in 2007 [16,17] and in 2017 the program was extended to include beta thalassemia major and hemoglobin H disease [18,19].

An inquiry performed in 2002 resulted in the estimation of 50 sickle cell patients born annually and at least 800 SCD patients in total [20]. The total number of SCD patients, adults and children, in The Netherlands is now estimated to be in an order of 1500–2000. This number is based on expert opinion only, but clinicians and researchers are working together to set up a national registry.

NBS for hemoglobinopathies is universal, i.e., without any preselection on the basis of the putative ethnic origin of the baby. The method of choice to analyze dried blood spots is HPLC. A distinctive feature of the Dutch program is that there is no second-tier method in place. Children with positive screening tests are referred to pediatric hematologists for confirmation. In spite of this practice, only five false positives were reported in the first 10 years of screening. Almost all of these false positives were carriers of HbS or had another hemoglobinopathy. The first year of screening resulted in 40 diagnoses of SCD [21]. The 2016 annual bulletin reported 30 referrals for SCD and 30 referrals for alpha and beta thalassemia combined (https://www.rivm.nl/sites/default/files/2018-11/HielprikMon2016-Engels-def.pdf). In addition 800–850 carriers are detected every year [22]. The carrier state is reported routinely to the general practitioner to facilitate family testing if parents do not object to knowing the carrier status of their child.

4. Spain

A national universal newborn screening program has been available in Spain since 1978. It is on a voluntary basis, but has a nearly 100% coverage. Universal screening for hemoglobinopathies started in the Madrid region in 2003, in the Basque country in 2011, in Valencia in 2012, and was extended nationwide in 2015. More than 400,000 neonates were screened in 2016 with 48 cases of SCD identified [23]. HPLC is the first test used in most of the regions. Confirmatory testing is done with HPLC on the same dried blood spot and on a new capillary sample before the age of three months.

5. Belgium

Belgium does not screen for hemoglobinopathies on a national level. However, there are currently three regional programs in place [24]. The *Cliniques Universitaires de Bruxelles, hôpital Erasme* (currently the LHUB-ULB) are responsible for the Brussels region. They were the first institutions to introduce NBS for SCD in Belgium in 1994 [25–28] and the only institutions to receive public funding until 2015.

Both of the other two screening projects are located in Liège at the *Centre Hospitalier Régional de la Citadelle* (CHR Citadelle), which started NBS for SCD solely in its own institution in 2002 [27] and the *Centre Hospitalier Universitaire de Liège* (CHU de Liège) that covers 14 maternity wards in Wallonia since 2007 [29,30]. SCD screening in the Liège region has a quasi-official status, but is not reimbursed by the insurance companies. It is financed through hospital funding.

Since 2008, Belgium has been running a registry for SCD patients. From the academic point-of-view it is interesting that all patients diagnosed with SCD in Belgium are reported to this registry. While some of them have been identified through NBS, others have been identified later in life on the basis of clinical symptoms. By comparing the two populations, the Belgian group was able to demonstrate that NBS for SCD improves clinical outcome by a significant reduction of bacteremia and hospitalization [31,32].

To complement the screening data from the well-established programs in Brussels and Liège, two thirds (n = 39,599) of all Belgian newborns were screened in a six-month pilot study [24]. The highest incidences were found in urban areas. However, in total, SCD was more common than any other target disease in the Belgian NBS program. 17 babies (1:2329) were diagnosed with sickling disorders. 1 in 77 was demonstrated to be heterozygous for hemoglobin S.

In terms of the methodology, the Belgian programs are heterogenous. While LHUB-ULB and CHR Citadelle used to screen by CE from liquid cord blood, CHU de Liège applied tandem mass spectrometry to dried blood spots on heel prick filter paper. HPLC and molecular genetics are used as confirmatory methods. In the pilot study, dried blood spots were examined by capillary electrophoresis. Positive results were confirmed by either HPLC or IEF. All Belgian projects have in common that all newborns were screened without any preselection on the basis of their putative ethnic origin (i.e., universal screening).

6. Italy

A National Newborn Screening Program (NBS) has been present in Italy since the nineties and around 500,000 babies are born every year. The National Health System is organized on a regional basis and, therefore, every region can organize its own NBS. Therefore, there are significant differences in the regional legislations regulating NBS and in the development of the regional NBS programs in terms of the diseases to be included, funding allocated and program organization (http://www.aismme.org/images/Linee_guida_05.08.pdf). The screening is mandatory but does not include hemoglobinopathies. Nevertheless, since the end of 2000, due to the increase of patients with SCD as a result of immigration, several scientific societies have started to raise the issue of NBS for SCD: the Italian Association of Pediatric Hematology Oncology (AIEOP) highly recommended NBS for SCD in its guidelines published in 2012 in Italian and 2013 in English [33] and in 2017 the AIEOP together with the Italian Society of Thalassemia and Hemoglobinopathies (SITE) issued a joint document for the recommendation of NBS for SCD in Italy (http://www.site-italia.org/file/collana_scientifica/libretto_5_2017/index.php). These efforts have led to the development of six NBS pilot programs [34–39], three of which are currently active [35,38,39] and one is being scaled up [37]. Two programs are universal [37,39] and the remaining are targeted [35]; one is antenatal. Methodologies and techniques vary: some use cord blood, others dried blood spot, HPLC is usually the first test whilst the confirmatory test can be molecular biology or IEF. Overall, the results of the universal programs are in line with those of other European countries with high immigration, with 1.16% incidence of positive tests (0.07% with SCD, 0.68% with sickle cell trait) [37].

7. Germany

NBS in Germany started in 1969 with nationwide testing of all newborns for phenylketonuria. Over the years, the number of targeted diseases rose to 16 with cystic fibrosis and tyrosinemia being the last implemented in 2016 and 2017, respectively. All target diseases are endocrine or metabolic disorders. NBS in Germany is offered to every family, but participation is voluntary. However, coverage is very close to 100%. In 2015, 737,575 babies were born in Germany and 539 confirmed diagnoses of NBS target diseases were made (1:1368).

SCD is not a target disease of the German NBS program. Principally, this is owing to the fact that the disease has not been endemic in Germany in the past. It has thus been neglected over decades, although a significant and steady increase of diagnoses was observed by Kohne and Kleihauer as early as in the late 1960s [40,41]. The first systematic attempt to identify newborns suffering from SCD was made by Genzel who started a targeted pilot project in her Department of Obstetrics in Munich [42]. One affected baby was diagnosed in a targeted screening approach of 306 children born to Sub-Saharan African mothers.

With the formation of the *GPOH-Konsortium Sichelzellkrankheit* and its official assignment by the German Society for Pediatric Oncology and Hematology (GPOH) to develop a management program for children and adolescents with SCD, awareness and care improved dramatically. To date, members of this consortium have completed four regional pilot studies on NBS for SCD [43–47]. Two have been done in the Berlin NBS laboratory and one in the Hamburg and the Heidelberg NBS laboratory, respectively. Another study in Berlin is currently recruiting patients and a joint German–Polish pilot project has recently been started.

Altogether, dried blood spot samples of 118,019 newborns have been investigated in the four published studies and 32 affected babies (1:3688) were identified as having SCD. These results led the authors to the conclusion that NBS for SCD is clearly indicated in Germany.

The formal application to introduce NBS for SCD was assessed by the *Gemeinsamer Bundesausschuss* (GBA) in May 2018 for the first time. The GBA is the political body that decides what the public health insurance companies have to pay for. It consists of representatives of the different interest groups in the German healthcare system (e.g., patients, doctors, insurance companies etc.). The GBA has admitted the application for the highly formal decision-making process. A result is not expected before May 2021.

8. Ireland

Ireland has had a national NBS program since 1966, for metabolic and endocrine diseases using heel prick and dried blood spot analysis. Participation is mandatory but opting out is possible.

Currently the program captures 99.9% of all newborn infants. Targeted and voluntary national hemoglobinopathy screening has been available since 2003. Currently, it is performed on cord blood using CE as first line testing and HPLC/IEF as a confirmatory test [48]. The number of newborns diagnosed by NBS with SCD or beta thalassemia major is 10–15/year and all are referred to a single pediatric hemoglobinopathy center.

9. Malta

In Malta, all newborn are screened for SCD (universal NBS program). In 2017, 4370 babies were tested, none of which suffered from the disorder. However, eight carriers were detected. As in many other countries, a two-tier strategy is applied. IEF serves as the first tier method. Any sample containing Hb S (i.e., heterozygous, homozygous or compound heterozygous, respectively) is re-examined by HPLC to confirm the first-tier result. In case of a positive result, the screening laboratory notifies the thalassemia and sickle cell clinic who in turn will notify the parents and an appointment is given for a follow up. If requested, parents and siblings are screened (personal communication).

10. Closing Remarks

Despite all these varieties, there is broad consensus among European NBS and SCD experts on the fundamental standards that a state-of-the-art NBS program for SCD should fulfil. These standards have recently been defined in a two-day consensus conference of more than 50 experts from 13 European countries and published elsewhere [49,50]. Future intensification of this collaboration will hopefully lead to a harmonization of NBS programs for SCD in Europe.

Funding: This research received no external funding.

Conflicts of Interest: The authors declare no conflict of interest.

References

1. National Sickle Cell Anemia Control Act. Available online: https://www.govinfo.gov/content/pkg/STATUTE-86/pdf/STATUTE-86-Pg136-2.pdf (accessed on 9 February 2019).
2. Gaston, M.H.; Verter, J.I.; Woods, G.; Pegelow, C.; Kelleher, J.; Presbury, G.; Zarkowsky, H.; Vichinsky, E.; Iyer, R.; Lobel, J.S.; et al. Prophylaxis with oral penicillin in children with sickle cell anemia. A randomized trial. *N. Engl. J. Med.* **1986**, *314*, 1593–1599. [CrossRef] [PubMed]
3. Zeuner, D.; Ades, A.E.; Karnon, J.; Brown, J.; Dezateux, C.; Anionwu, E.N. Antenatal and neonatal haemoglobinopathy screening in the UK: Review and economic analysis. *Health Technol. Assess.* **1999**, *3*, 1–186.
4. *The NHS Plan: A Plan for Investment, A Plan for Reform*; Department of Health: London, UK, 2000.
5. Moat, S.J.; Rees, D.; King, L.; Ifederu, A.; Harvey, K.; Hall, K.; Lloyd, G.; Morrell, C.; Hillier, S. Newborn blood spot screening for sickle cell disease by using tandem mass spectrometry: Implementation of a protocol to identify only the disease states of sickle cell disease. *Clin. Chem.* **2014**, *60*, 373–380. [CrossRef] [PubMed]
6. Streetly, A.; Sisodia, R.; Dick, M.; Latinovic, R.; Hounsell, K.; Dormandy, E. Evaluation of newborn sickle cell screening programme in England: 2010-2016. *Arch. Dis Child.* **2018**, *103*, 648–653. [CrossRef] [PubMed]
7. Daniel, Y.; Henthorn, J. *Tandem Mass Spectrometry for Sickle Cell and Thalassaemia Newborn Screening Pilot Study*; Public Health England: London, UK, 2015.
8. Daniel, Y.A.; Henthorn, J. Newborn screening for sickling and other haemoglobin disorders using tandem mass spectrometry: A pilot study of methodology in laboratories in England. *J. Med. Screen.* **2016**, *23*, 175–178. [CrossRef] [PubMed]
9. Daniel, Y.; Henthorn, J. Reliability of the current newborn screening action value for beta thalassaemia disease detection in England: A prospective study. *J. Med. Screen.* **2018**. [CrossRef] [PubMed]
10. Streetly, A.; Latinovic, R.; Henthorn, J.; Daniel, Y.; Dormandy, E.; Darbyshire, P.; Mantio, D.; Fraser, L.; Farrar, L.; Will, A.; et al. Newborn bloodspot results: Predictive value of screen positive test for thalassaemia major. *J. Med. Screen* **2013**, *20*, 183–187. [CrossRef] [PubMed]

11. Saint-Martin, C.; Romana, M.; Bibrac, A.; Brudey, K.; Tarer, V.; Divialle-Doumdo, L.; Petras, M.; Keclard-Christophe, L.; Lamothe, S.; Broquere, C.; et al. Universal newborn screening for haemoglobinopathies in Guadeloupe (French West Indies): A 27-year experience. *J. Med. Screen.* **2013**, *20*, 177–182. [CrossRef] [PubMed]
12. Bardakdjian-Michau, J.; Bahuau, M.; Hurtrel, D.; Godart, C.; Riou, J.; Mathis, M.; Goossens, M.; Badens, C.; Ducrocq, R.; Elion, J.; et al. Neonatal screening for sickle cell disease in France. *J. Clin. Pathol.* **2009**, *62*, 31–33. [CrossRef] [PubMed]
13. Thuret, I.; Sarles, J.; Merono, F.; Suzineau, E.; Collomb, J.; Lena-Russo, D.; Levy, N.; Bardakdjian, J.; Badens, C. Neonatal screening for sickle cell disease in France: Evaluation of the selective process. *J. Clin. Pathol.* **2010**, *63*, 548–551. [CrossRef] [PubMed]
14. Bardakdjian-Michau, J.; Guilloud-Bataille, M.; Maier-Redelsperger, M.; Elion, J.; Girot, R.; Feingold, J.; Galacteros, F.; de Montalembert, M. Decreased morbidity in homozygous sickle cell disease detected at birth. *Hemoglobin* **2002**, *26*, 211–217. [CrossRef] [PubMed]
15. Couque, N.; Girard, D.; Ducrocq, R.; Boizeau, P.; Haouari, Z.; Missud, F.; Holvoet, L.; Ithier, G.; Belloy, M.; Odievre, M.H.; et al. Improvement of medical care in a cohort of newborns with sickle-cell disease in North Paris: Impact of national guidelines. *Br. J. Haematol.* **2016**, *173*, 927–937. [CrossRef] [PubMed]
16. Bouva, M.J.; Mohrmann, K.; Brinkman, H.B.; Kemper-Proper, E.A.; Elvers, B.; Loeber, J.G.; Verheul, F.E.; Giordano, P.C. Implementing neonatal screening for haemoglobinopathies in the Netherlands. *J. Med. Screen.* **2010**, *17*, 58–65. [CrossRef] [PubMed]
17. *Neonatal Screening*; Health Council of the Netherlands: The Hague, The Netherlands, 2005.
18. Bouva, M.J.; Sollaino, C.; Perseu, L.; Galanello, R.; Giordano, P.C.; Harteveld, C.L.; Cnossen, M.H.; Schielen, P.C.; Elvers, L.H.; Peters, M. Relationship between neonatal screening results by HPLC and the number of alpha-thalassaemia gene mutations; consequences for the cut-off value. *J. Med. Screen.* **2011**, *18*, 182–186. [CrossRef] [PubMed]
19. *Neonatal Screening: New Recommendations*; Health Council of the Netherlands: The Hague, The Netherlands, 2015.
20. Giordano, P.C.; Bouva, M.J.; Harteveld, C.L. A confidential inquiry estimating the number of patients affected with sickle cell disease and thalassemia major confirms the need for a prevention strategy in the Netherlands. *Hemoglobin* **2004**, *28*, 287–296. [CrossRef] [PubMed]
21. Peter, M.; Appel, I.M.; Cnossen, M.H.; Breuning-Boers, J.M.; Heijboer, H. Sickle cell disease in heel prick screening. I. *Ned. Tijdschr. Geneeskd.* **2009**, *153*, 854–857.
22. Vansenne, F.; de Borgie, C.; Bouva, M.J.; Legdeur, M.A.; van Zwieten, R.; Petrij, F.; Peters, M. Sickle cell disease in heel prick screening. II. *Ned. Tijdschr. Geneeskd.* **2009**, *153*, 858–861. [PubMed]
23. Cela, E.; Bellon, J.M.; de la Cruz, M.; Belendez, C.; Berrueco, R.; Ruiz, A.; Elorza, I.; Diaz de Heredia, C.; Cervera, A.; Valles, G.; et al. National registry of hemoglobinopathies in Spain (REPHem). *Pediatr. Blood Cancer* **2017**, *64*. [CrossRef] [PubMed]
24. Ketelslegers, O.; Eyskens, F.; Boemer, F.; Bours, V.; Minon, J.-M.; Gulbis, B. Epidemiological data on sickle cell disease in Belgium. *Belg. J. Hematol.* **2015**, *6*, 135–141.
25. Gulbis, B.; Tshilolo, L.; Cotton, F.; Lin, C.; Vertongen, F. Newborn screening for haemoglobinopathies: The Brussels experience. *J. Med. Screen.* **1999**, *6*, 11–15. [CrossRef] [PubMed]
26. Gulbis, B.; Ferster, A.; Cotton, F.; Lebouchard, M.P.; Cochaux, P.; Vertongen, F. Neonatal haemoglobinopathy screening: Review of a 10-year programme in Brussels. *J. Med. Screen.* **2006**, *13*, 76–78. [CrossRef] [PubMed]
27. Gulbis, B.; Cotton, F.; Ferster, A.; Ketelslegers, O.; Dresse, M.F.; Ronge-Collard, E.; Minon, J.M.; Le, P.Q.; Vertongen, F. Neonatal haemoglobinopathy screening in Belgium. *J. Clin. Pathol.* **2009**, *62*, 49–52. [CrossRef] [PubMed]
28. Wolff, F.; Cotton, F.; Gulbis, B. Screening for haemoglobinopathies on cord blood: Laboratory and clinical experience. *J. Med. Screen.* **2012**, *19*, 116–122. [CrossRef] [PubMed]
29. Boemer, F.; Cornet, Y.; Libioulle, C.; Segers, K.; Bours, V.; Schoos, R. 3-years experience review of neonatal screening for hemoglobin disorders using tandem mass spectrometry. *Clin. Chim. Acta* **2011**, *412*, 1476–1479. [CrossRef] [PubMed]
30. Boemer, F.; Ketelslegers, O.; Minon, J.M.; Bours, V.; Schoos, R. Newborn screening for sickle cell disease using tandem mass spectrometry. *Clin. Chem.* **2008**, *54*, 2036–2041. [CrossRef] [PubMed]

31. Le, P.Q.; Ferster, A.; Cotton, F.; Vertongen, F.; Vermylen, C.; Vanderfaeillie, A.; Dedeken, L.; Heijmans, C.; Ketelslegers, O.; Dresse, M.F.; et al. Sickle cell disease from Africa to Belgium, from neonatal screening to clinical management. *Med. Trop.* **2010**, *70*, 467–470.
32. Le, P.Q.; Ferster, A.; Dedeken, L.; Vermylen, C.; Vanderfaeillie, A.; Rozen, L.; Heijmans, C.; Huybrechts, S.; Devalck, C.; Cotton, F.; et al. Neonatal screening improves sickle cell disease clinical outcome in Belgium. *J. Med. Screen.* **2017**, *25*, 57–63. [CrossRef] [PubMed]
33. Colombatti, R.; Perrotta, S.; Samperi, P.; Casale, M.; Masera, N.; Palazzi, G.; Sainati, L.; Russo, G.; Italian Association of Pediatric Hematology-Oncology Sickle Cell Disease Working Group. Organizing national responses for rare blood disorders: The Italian experience with sickle cell disease in childhood. *Orphanet J. Rare Dis.* **2013**, *8*, 169. [CrossRef] [PubMed]
34. Rolla, R.; Castagno, M.; Zaffaroni, M.; Grigollo, B.; Colombo, S.; Piccotti, S.; Dellora, C.; Bona, G.; Bellomo, G. Neonatal screening for sickle cell disease and other hemoglobinopathies in "the changing Europe". *Clin. Lab.* **2014**, *60*, 2089–2093. [CrossRef] [PubMed]
35. Venturelli, D.; Lodi, M.; Palazzi, G.; Bergonzini, G.; Doretto, G.; Zini, A.; Monica, C.; Cano, M.C.; Ilaria, M.; Montagnani, G.; et al. Sickle cell disease in areas of immigration of high-risk populations: A low cost and reproducible method of screening in northern Italy. *Blood Transfus.* **2014**, *12*, 346–351. [CrossRef] [PubMed]
36. Ballardini, E.; Tarocco, A.; Marsella, M.; Bernardoni, R.; Carandina, G.; Melandri, C.; Guerra, G.; Patella, A.; Zucchelli, M.; Ferlini, A.; et al. Universal neonatal screening for sickle cell disease and other haemoglobinopathies in Ferrara, Italy. *Blood Transfus.* **2013**, *11*, 245–249. [CrossRef] [PubMed]
37. Martella, M.; Cattaneo, L.; Viola, G.; Azzena, S.; Cappellari, A.; Baraldi, E.; Zorloni, C.; Masera, N.; Biondi, A.; Basso, G.; et al. Universal Newborn Screening for Sickle Cell Disease: Preliminary Results of the First Year of a Multicentric Italian Project. In Proceedings of the 22nd Annual Congress of the European Hematology Association, Madrid, spain, June 2017; pp. 22–25.
38. De Zen, L.; Dall'Amico, R.; Sainati, L.; Colombatti, R.; Testa, E.R.; Catapano, R.; Zanolli, F. Screening neonatale per le emoglobinopatie su Dried Blood Spot. In Proceedings of the XXXVI. Congresso Nazionale Associazione Italiana Ematologia Oncologia Pediatrica (AIEOP), Pisa, Italy, June 2010; pp. 6–8.
39. Mandrile, G.; Cavazzuti, C.; Gaglioti, C.M.; Cociglio, S.; Lux, C.M.; Chiavilli, F.; Piga, A. 40 anni di screening delle emoglobinopatie: l'esperienza di Rovigo. In Proceedings of the X. Congresso Nazionale SITE, Rome, Italy, September 2018; pp. 27–29.
40. Kohne, E.; Kleihauer, E. Häufigkeit und Formen von anomalen Hämoglobinen und Thalassämie-Syndromen in der deutschen Bevölkerung. *Klinische Wochenschrift* **1974**, *52*, 1003–1010. [CrossRef]
41. Kohne, E.; Kleihauer, E. Hemoglobinopathies: A longitudinal study over four decades. *Dtsch. Arztebl. Int.* **2010**, *107*, 65–71. [CrossRef] [PubMed]
42. Dickerhoff, R.; Genzel-Boroviczeny, O.; Kohne, E. Haemoglobinopathies and newborn haemoglobinopathy screening in Germany. *J. Clin. Pathol.* **2009**, *62*, 34. [CrossRef] [PubMed]
43. Lobitz, S.; Klein, J.; Brose, A.; Blankenstein, O.; Frommel, C. Newborn screening by tandem mass spectrometry confirms the high prevalence of sickle cell disease among German newborns. *Ann. Hematol.* **2018**. [CrossRef] [PubMed]
44. Lobitz, S.; Frommel, C.; Brose, A.; Klein, J.; Blankenstein, O. Incidence of sickle cell disease in an unselected cohort of neonates born in Berlin, Germany. *Eur. J. Hum. Genet.* **2014**, *22*, 1051–1053. [CrossRef] [PubMed]
45. Frommel, C.; Brose, A.; Klein, J.; Blankenstein, O.; Lobitz, S. Newborn screening for sickle cell disease: Technical and legal aspects of a German pilot study with 38,220 participants. *BioMed Res. Int.* **2014**, *2014*, 695828. [CrossRef] [PubMed]

46. Kunz, J.B.; Awad, S.; Happich, M.; Muckenthaler, L.; Lindner, M.; Gramer, G.; Okun, J.G.; Hoffmann, G.F.; Bruckner, T.; Muckenthaler, M.U.; et al. Significant prevalence of sickle cell disease in Southwest Germany: Results from a birth cohort study indicate the necessity for newborn screening. *Ann. Hematol.* **2016**, *95*, 397–402. [CrossRef] [PubMed]
47. Grosse, R.; Lukacs, Z.; Cobos, P.N.; Oyen, F.; Ehmen, C.; Muntau, B.; Timmann, C.; Noack, B. The Prevalence of Sickle Cell Disease and Its Implication for Newborn Screening in Germany (Hamburg Metropolitan Area). *Pediatr. Blood Cancer* **2015**. [CrossRef] [PubMed]
48. Gibbons, C.; Geoghegan, R.; Conroy, H.; Lippacott, S.; O'Brien, D.; Lynam, P.; Langabeer, L.; Cotter, M.; Smith, O.; McMahon, C. Sickle cell disease: Time for a targeted neonatal screening programme. *Ir. Med. J.* **2015**, *108*, 43–45. [PubMed]
49. Shook, L.M.; Ware, R.E. Sickle cell screening in Europe: The time has come. *Br. J. Haematol.* **2018**, *183*, 534–535. [CrossRef] [PubMed]
50. Lobitz, S.; Telfer, P.; Cela, E.; Allaf, B.; Angastiniotis, M.; Backman Johansson, C.; Badens, C.; Bento, C.; Bouva, M.J.; Canatan, D.; et al. Newborn screening for sickle cell disease in Europe: Recommendations from a Pan-European Consensus Conference. *Br. J. Haematol.* **2018**, *183*, 648–660. [CrossRef] [PubMed]

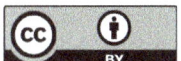 © 2019 by the authors. Licensee MDPI, Basel, Switzerland. This article is an open access article distributed under the terms and conditions of the Creative Commons Attribution (CC BY) license (http://creativecommons.org/licenses/by/4.0/).

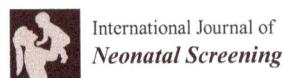 International Journal of
Neonatal Screening

Article

Neonatal Screening for Sickle Cell Disease in Belgium for More than 20 Years: An Experience for Comprehensive Care Improvement

Béatrice Gulbis [1,*], Phu-Quoc Lê [2], Olivier Ketelslegers [3], Marie-Françoise Dresse [4], Anne-Sophie Adam [1], Frédéric Cotton [1], François Boemer [5], Vincent Bours [5], Jean-Marc Minon [3] and Alina Ferster [2]

1. Department of Clinical Chemistry, LHUB-ULB, Université Libre de Bruxelles (ULB) 322, Rue Haute, 1000 Brussels, Belgium; AnneSophie.Adam@LHUB-ULB.be (A.-S.A.); Frederic.Cotton@LHUB-ULB.be (F.C.)
2. Department of Hemato-Oncology Hôpital Universitaire des Enfants Reine Fabiola, Université Libre de Bruxelles (ULB) 15, av. J.J. Crocq, 1020 Brussels, Belgium; phuquoc.le@huderf.be (P.-Q.L.); alina.ferster@huderf.be (A.F.)
3. Department of Laboratory Medicine CHR de la Citadelle, 1, Boulevard de la 12ème Ligne, 4000 Liège, Belgium; olivier.ketelslegers@chrcitadelle.be (O.K.); jean.marc.minon@chrcitadelle.be (J.-M.M.)
4. Department of Pediatric, University Hospital Liège, CHR de la Citadelle, 1, Boulevard de la 12ème Ligne, 4000 Liège, Belgium; marie.francoise.dresse@chrcitadelle.be
5. Department of Human Genetics CHU Sart Tilman, Université de Liège (ULg) Domaine Universitaire du Sart Tilmant Bâtiment 35-B, 4000 Liège, Belgium; F.Boemer@chuliege.be (F.B.); vbours@chuliege.be (V.B.)

* Correspondence: Beatrice.Gulbis@LHUB-ULB.be; Tel.: +32-2-555-34-27; Fax: +32-2-555-66-55

Received: 7 October 2018; Accepted: 20 November 2018; Published: 27 November 2018

Abstract: Our previous results reported that compared to sickle cell patients who were not screened at birth, those who benefited from it had a lower incidence of a first bacteremia and a reduced number and days of hospitalizations. In this context, this article reviews the Belgian experience on neonatal screening for sickle cell disease (SCD). It gives an update on the two regional neonatal screening programs for SCD in Belgium and their impact on initiatives to improve clinical care for sickle cell patients. Neonatal screening in Brussels and Liège Regions began in 1994 and 2002, respectively. Compiled results for the 2009 to 2017 period demonstrated a birth prevalence of sickle cell disorder above 1:2000. In parallel, to improve clinical care, (1) a committee of health care providers dedicated to non-malignant hematological diseases has been created within the Belgian Haematology Society; (2) a clinical registry was implemented in 2008 and has been updated in 2018; (3) a plan of action has been proposed to the Belgian national health authority. To date, neonatal screening is not integrated into the respective Belgian regional neonatal screening programs, the ongoing initiatives in Brussels and Liège Regions are not any further funded and better management of the disease through the implementation of specific actions is not yet perceived as a public health priority in Belgium.

Keywords: sickle cell disease; neonatal screening program; registry; birth prevalence

1. Introduction

At the World Health Organization, sickle cell disease has been recognized as a global public health problem [1]. The different migratory flows of recent decades have influenced the disease in European countries and in particular in Belgium [2]. According to our survey in 2007, there were approximately 400 patients (0.0036% of the total population) with sickle cell disease (SCD) living in Belgium. The implementation of a Belgian registry for SCD in 2008 allowed us to demonstrate that at the end of 2012, 469 SCD patients were regularly followed and registered by eight Belgian hospitals [3].

The benefit of neonatal screening for SCD has been established for many years [4]. Birth prevalence of this disease is not the only criterion for choosing to include sickle cell disease in the neonatal screening program, but in countries where birth prevalence of the condition is greater than 1:6000, this has been shown to be cost-effective [5]. However, in several European countries such as Belgium, neonatal screening for SCD is not part of the national neonatal screening program. Indeed, in Belgium, there are no national recommendations for sickle cell disease screening at birth and only local initiatives offer the benefit of early diagnosis to a small number of families. Following a successful Belgian screening in 2013 for two-thirds of neonates performed as part of a pilot study, it has been shown that the birth prevalence of SCD was 1:2329 [6].

In this context, this paper gives an update on the neonatal screening results for SCD and overall hemoglobinopathies in two different Belgian regions. In parallel with the increase in the number of sickle cell neonates born in Belgium, it also highlights the initiatives that have been conducted to improve the clinical care program.

2. Material and Methods

2.1. Neonatal Screening for Sickle Cell Disease

Neonatal screening for SCD began in five Brussels maternity wards in December 1994, but has been offered to all neonates in all maternity wards of the Brussels Region since 2004 (2004–2017: 310,053 neonates screened); screening began in one maternity ward in Liège Region in 2002 and was extended to 15 maternity wards in Liège Region in 2009 (East of Belgium; 2008–2017: 186,829 neonates screened). It is realized in three screening centers i.e., Brussels University Laboratory (LHUB-ULB), Centre Hospitalier Régional (CHR) de la Citadelle and Centre Hospitalier Universitaire (CHU) du Sart Tilman. The neonatal screening process is described in Table 1 and has been detailed previously [7–9]. Briefly, in LHUB-ULB and CHR de la Citadelle, liquid umbilical cord blood samples in EDTA were screened initially using an isoelectric focusing technique (IEF) (Perkin Elmer Life Sciences, Zaventem, Belgium) and since 2008, using a capillary zone electrophoresis (CZE) technique (Sebia Benelux, Vilvoorde, Belgium) [6]. In CHU du Sart Tilman, heel prick samples on filter paper were screened by tandem mass spectrometry (TMS) [7,8]. If a hemoglobin variant is detected, further analysis is performed on the same sample using high performance liquid chromatography (BioRad, Hercules, CA, USA) or DNA analysis [7–9]. If confirmed, a new sample is requested to use as a control.

Table 1. Neonatal screening process (offered to all neonates). CHR = Centre Hospitalier Régional. IEF = isoelectric focusing. CZE = capillary zone electrophoresis. TMS = tandem mass spectrometry.

Screening Centre	Sample	First Screening Test	Confirmation Test (Same Sample)	Report of Results	Ref.
Brussels Region	Umbilical cord blood liquid	IEF (<2008) CZE (≥2008)	HPLC	Any hemoglobinopathy detected	[7]
CHR Citadelle	Umbilical cord blood liquid	CZE	HPLC	Any hemoglobinopathy detected	[8]
Liège Region	Heel prick/filter paper	TMS	DNA	Any hemoglobinopathy detected	[9]

For the three screening centers, reports of results concern all SCD and all minor and major forms of hemoglobinopathy detected by the technique (Table 1). The screening of SCD in a neonate is reported immediately to the local coordinator and the medical staff of the maternity ward concerned. A new sample is requested for diagnosis.

For clarity, all results were also compiled in one period, i.e., 2009 to 2017, that allows us to report all results obtained from the three screening centers.

After confirmation of sickle cell disease on a new sample and, if feasible, before leaving the maternity ward, the families of an affected neonate received counselling and were referred to a specialized healthcare center where an initial visit was scheduled. The reference centers ensured the monitoring of affected children. The comprehensive care program includes the education of the patient and parents on subjects such as the prevention of complications, lifestyle, and management of fever and pain. The priority is to offer comprehensive and integrated care from neonatal screening throughout childhood and beyond to prevent acute complications, to delay the onset of chronic organ damage, and to treat acute complications for all neonates diagnosed with SCD. It is coordinated by a pediatrician who has acquired special skills in the care of patients with SCD.

2.2. Belgian Network of Health Care Providers and Registry for Sickle Cell Patients

In 2006, a red blood cell (RBC) disorders committee within a scientific society (the Belgian Haematology Society (BHS)) called the BHS RBC Committee was created. To date, it consists of 25 partners working in 14 different Belgian hospitals. The main objective of this network was to improve health care for patients affected by a non-malignant hematological disease, and in particular SCD. It does not currently benefit from any operating subsidy. It was supported on a temporary basis by grants. The main actors are pediatricians, adult hematologists, nurses and clinical biologists. To offer a unique tool to monitor the evolution of the population with SCD and to collect information on the main SCD complications (in particular for neonates screened at birth), a registry has been set up in 2008 by this committee. The objectives and implementation of the Belgian registry has been detailed previously [2]. Briefly, the BHS RBC Committee administers a centralized Belgian registry of patients with SCD. Eight centers participated with patient registration. Without national support, but thanks to a grant, in 2018, an updated registry has been launched and today, 12 centers participate. The items in the database were the subject of a consensus within the BHS RBC Committee. These data are updated annually. They make it possible to evaluate the benefit of neonatal screening and the follow-up of the patients screened at birth. For data privacy reasons, the information can only be accessed by healthcare professionals.

2.3. Comprehensive Care Improvement Plan

In 2014, to improve health care at a national level, the BHS RBC Committee proposed to define a plan of action. As part of the Belgian plan for rare diseases, this was submitted to the health authorities.

3. Results

3.1. Neonatal Screening for Sickle Cell Disease

During 2009 to 2017, 396,894 neonates were screened. This represents approximately 33% of births in Belgium. Screening coverage is almost 100%, except in two Brussels maternity wards where it is 85%. Birth prevalence of SCD and likely heterozygosity for hemoglobin (Hb) S are reported in Table 2. One sickle cell child born in one of the maternity wards where screening is performed was reported as not having been screened i.e., FSD^{Punjab}. The maternity ward has a screening coverage of around 85%. Most of the patients are homozygous for Hb S or compound heterozygous for Hb S and beta-thalassemia (210/246); 27/246 patients had a Hb SC disease.

Table 2. Distribution by year of neonates screened as having a sickle cell disease (SCD) i.e., homozygous for Hb S, compound heterozygous for Hb S and β-thalassemia, Hb C or another Hb variant; or likely heterozygous for hemoglobin S (FAS).

Year	Neonates Screened All Regions (n)	SCD Both Regions (n)	SCD Both Regions Birth Prevalence	FAS Brussels Region (n)	FAS Brussels Region Birth Prevalence	FAS Liège Region (n)	FAS Liège Region Birth Prevalence
2009	40,026	25	1:1601	421	1:54	159	1:109
2010	40,579	25	1:1561	449	1:52	150	1:115
2011	40,262	36	1:1088	458	1:50	112	1:154
2012	40,675	24	1:1768	460	1:51	175	1:98
2013	40,241	22	1:1829	520	1:45	161	1:104
2014	40,144	28	1:1487	447	1:52	192	1:87
2015	39,748	27	1:1529	449	1:52	174	1:94
2016	39,292	25	1:1572	504	1:46	200	1:82
2017	37,364	35	1:1068	503	1:42	193	1:83
Total	358,331	251	1:1427	4211	1:49	1516	1:100

The highest birth prevalence of neonates likely heterozygous for Hb S were observed for the two most recent years in both Brussels and Liège regions (Table 2). It is the most frequent hemoglobin variant observed in both regions that offer screening for SCD, with the most prevalent sickle cell disease being homozygosity for Hb S; β-thalassemia was observed only for two and seven neonates in the Brussels and Liège regions, respectively (Table 3).

Table 3. Neonatal screening for SCD by region: 2009–2017.

Type	Birth Prevalence Brussels Region n = 206,984	Birth Prevalence Liège Region n = 151,347
FS	1:1522	1:2481
FSC	1:7666	1:16,816
FSX	1:68,995	-
FE	-	1:151,347
FC	1:34,497	1:21,621
F-	1:103,492	1:21,621
FAS	1:49	1:100
FAC	1:394	1:655
FAE	1:2275	1:2259
FAD *	1:2587	1:7567
FAO *	1:4600	1:75,674

* Variant not screened by the method used in Centre Hospitalier Universitaire de Liège before 2014. Neonates homozygous for Hb S or compound heterozygous for Hb S and β-thalassemia (FS) or compound heterozygous for Hb S and C (FSC) or another Hb variant (FSX). Neonates homozygous for Hb C or compound heterozygous for Hb C and β-thalassemia (FC). Neonates homozygous for Hb E or compound heterozygous for Hb CE and β-thalassemia (FE). Neonates with absence of Hb A (F-). Neonates likely heterozygous for a hemoglobin variant i.e., Hb S (FAS), Hb C (FAC), Hb E (FAE), Hb D-Punjab (FAD), Hb O-Arab (FAO).

3.2. Belgian Network of Health Care Providers and Registry for Sickle Cell Patients

At the end of 2012, 469 patients were registered in the Belgian registry of patients with SCD. In September 2018, 538 patients had been registered in the updated database; 285 were born in Belgium, of which 64% (182/285) benefited from the neonatal screening program for SCD and 53 did not (i.e., born in other regions than those covered by neonatal screening and at least one born in the Brussels region). Compared to data in 2012, this means a longer follow-up and an increase in the number of affected patients screened at birth (or not).

3.3. Comprehensive Care Improvement Plan

A plan of action to improve health care for SCD patients has been proposed and submitted to the National Institute of Health in 2014 (Figure 1). To date, only the recognition of SCD as a rare disease in Belgium (Step 1) through the recognition of reference centers for hemoglobinopathies (Step 4) at the Belgian and European levels i.e., Cliniques Universitaires de Bruxelles Hôpital Erasme, and one related department i.e., Department of Hemato-Oncology, Immunology and Transplantation—Hôpital Universitaire des Enfants Reine Fabiola, has been effective.

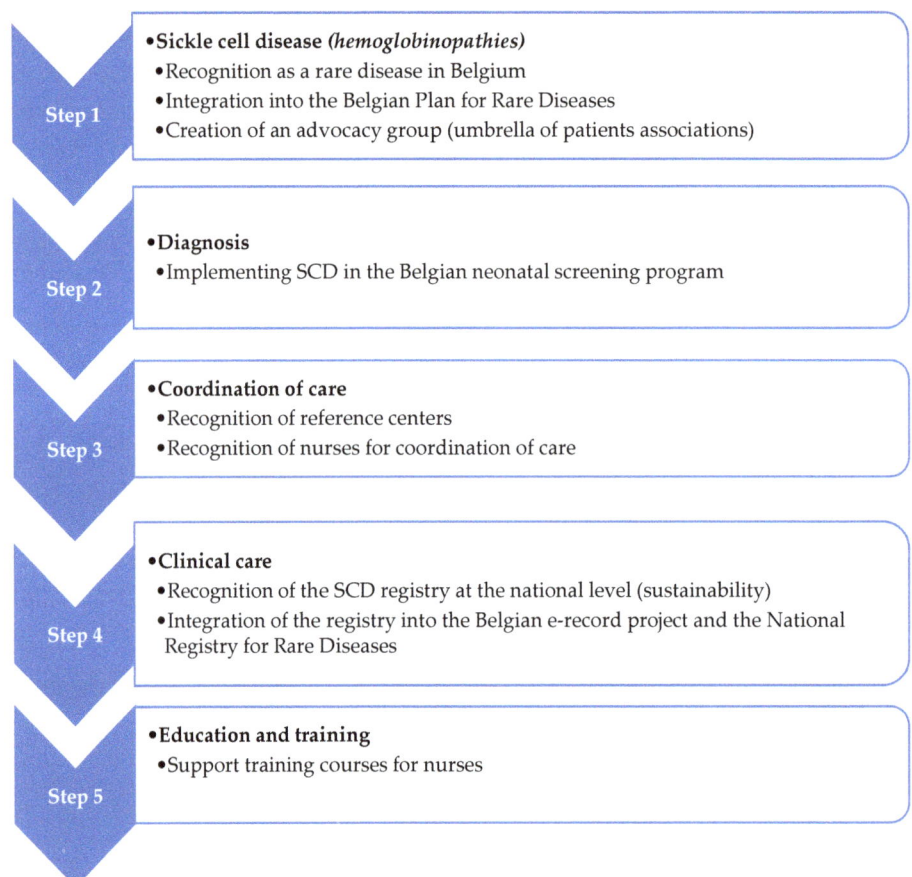

Figure 1. Plan of action to improve clinical care for SCD patients in Belgium.

The other steps of the plan (Figure 1) have not been debated or implemented. In particular, sickle cell disease has still not been included in the national neonatal screening program.

4. Discussion

Our study demonstrated that throughout the period of 2009 to 2017, the birth prevalence of sickle cell disease in two Belgian regions was higher than 1:2000 and heterozygosity for Hb S was the highest during the years 2016 and 2017 (>1:50 and >1:90 for Brussels and Liège Regions, respectively). To date, neonatal screening for SCD is not yet integrated into the national neonatal screening program. It also has no funding. Neonatal screening has been and is an important lever for providing health care improvements to sickle cell patients. In this respect, the creation of a Belgian network of health care professionals, particularly composed of many pediatricians, within a Belgian scientific society and the resulting initiatives (such as the implementation of a clinical registry of sickle cell patients) have been important steps. An action plan has also been proposed to the National Institute of Health in 2014.

In recent decades, as a result of migratory flows, the disease has spread throughout the world, particularly in Western Europe. It is therefore becoming a major concern of public health policies [10,11]. Belgium, with 20% of migrants including 12.5% of at-risk origin and its history of colonization in Africa and more particularly in the Democratic Republic of Congo, is also concerned [12]. During a pilot phase of neonatal screening extended over a period of six months and covering 2/3 of births in Belgium, the birth prevalence observed for SCD is 1/2329 [6]. This makes SCD one of the most common inherited diseases in Belgium, far more prevalent than other commonly screened disorders such as phenylketonuria. Birth prevalence of SCD remains at >1:2500 in regions were neonatal screening is performed. Despite the birth prevalence increases in 2016 and 2017 in the two regions where screening was performed, without national data, it is quite difficult to draw conclusions.

The advantage of neonatal screening in reducing early mortality is demonstrated in the US, various European countries and Jamaica. Vichinsky et al. showed that after a median follow-up of seven years, the overall mortality rate of patients diagnosed at birth was 1.8%, compared to 8% in children diagnosed after the age of three months [13]. Similarly, in the Jamaican cohort, less than 1% of children died in the first two years of life when preventive strategies were available, compared to 14% when early interventions could not be implemented [14]. In Brazil, however, the mortality rate of children with SCD remains high, at 7.4%, despite an effective, ongoing and comprehensive screening program. There are many reasons for this, including the low socio-economic and cultural status of affected families complicating regular clinical monitoring, long trips to health facilities, the short interval between onset of symptoms and death and inexperience of the health staff to recognize and manage SCD acute events [15]. Quinn et al. have demonstrated that neonatal screening minimizes morbidity and mortality through antibiotic prophylaxis and parental education [16,17]. Currently, with the addition of combined vaccination against pneumococcus and *Haemophilus influenzae* on the one hand, and integrated management that focuses on family education on the other hand, the mortality of newborns screened decreased to less than 1%. Screening is not widespread in Belgium, and in 2008, our BHS RBC Committee established a sickle cell registry. These two aspects allowed us to compare the future of SCD children that were screened (or not) at birth [18]. If we were unable to demonstrate a significant reduction in mortality among children screened in the neonatal period compared to those that were not, our previous results showed a benefit of neonatal screening in terms of decreasing the incidence of a first bacteremia and reducing the number and days of hospitalizations (expressed per 100 patient-years). Our only two deaths (in 1996 and 2000) occurred in very young patients, during a period marked by poor compliance and when integrated management was still immature [18]. Couque et al. also emphasized the importance of optimal adherence and integrated care on the prognosis of patients in 2016 [19]. The update of our cohort in the Belgian registry will allow us to monitor the effectiveness of the management of sickle cell patients and to provide any additional data regarding the benefit of screening.

The establishment of an integrated system for diagnosis and patient care is only beginning to emerge in Europe for several reasons. It concerns migrant minority communities of various origins, often isolated, disadvantaged and whose access to health care is not always easy; the perception of sickle cell disease in the communities concerned was not or is no longer adequate; and by lack of knowledge, the disease is often not recognized or trivialized by members of the medical community as well as by health managers [1]. In Belgium, a group of doctors involved in the management of sickle cell disease began in the early 2000s to reflect on the feasibility of an integrated care system initially in Brussels. This group wanted to focus on prevention while promoting health within a multidisciplinary group, as recommended by the World Health Organization [1]. This network aims to bring together all health professionals and patient associations concerned in a search for the best evidence of prevention, care and epidemiological data. It also aims to alert national health authorities to the real public health problems posed by SCD. This explains the approach that aims to propose an action plan for improving the management of SCD.

5. Conclusions

Neonatal screening for SCD performed in two Belgian regions demonstrated that its birth prevalence is higher than 1:2000. Those results pose the question of its integration into the regional neonatal screening program. In order to appreciate the benefit of neonatal screening in our care setting, a sickle cell registry has been set up and has been updated in 2018 with an increasing number of patients screened for ongoing evaluation. These initiatives have been one of the driving forces behind the creation of a Belgian network of healthcare professionals that aims to improve the management of all sickle cell patients.

Author Contributions: Methodology, B.G., O.K., F.B.; validation, P.-Q.L., A.F., F.C., F.B. and M.-F.D.; formal analysis, B.G., O.K., F.B., V.B., F.C., A.-S.A., P.-Q.L., A.F.; data curation, B.G., O.K., M.-F.D., J.-M.M., F.B., V.B., F.C., A.-S.A., P.-Q.L., A.F.; writing—original draft preparation, B.G.; writing—review and editing, P.-Q.L., O.K., M.-F.D., A.-S.A., F.C., F.B., V.B. and A.F.; funding acquisition, B.G., J.-M.M., V.B., A.F.

Funding: Neonatal screening for SCD was supported in the Brussels Region by a grant from "INAMI/RIZIV" from 2004 to 2015. The SCD registry was supported by grants from Novartis Pharma S.A.S. and "Iris-Recherche—N° 2017-J1820690-206899".

Acknowledgments: The authors would like to thank all caregivers who participated in the neonatal hemoglobinopathy screening program and the members of the Red Blood Cell Belgian Haematology Society committee for their fruitful collaboration.

Conflicts of Interest: The authors declare no conflict of interest.

References

1. Sickle cell anemia. Available online: http://apps.who.int/gb/archive/pdf_files/wha59/a59_9-en.pdf (accessed on 11 November 2018).
2. Aguilar Martinez, P.; Angastiniotis, M.; Eleftheriou, A.; Gulbis, B.; Mañú Pereira Mdel, M.; Petrova-Benedict, R.; Corrons, J.L. Haemoglobinopathies in Europe: Health & migration policy perspectives. *Orphanet J. Rare Dis.* **2014**, *9*, 97. [CrossRef] [PubMed]
3. Lê, P.Q.; Gulbis, B.; Dedeken, L.; Dupont, S.; Vanderfaeillie, A.; Heijmans, C.; Huybrechts, S.; Devalck, C.; Efira, A.; Dresse, M.F.; et al. Survival among children and adults with sickle cell disease in belgium: Benefit from hydroxyurea treatment. *Pediatr. Blood Cancer* **2015**, *62*, 1956–1961. [CrossRef] [PubMed]
4. Gaston, M.H.; Verter, J.I.; Woods, G.; Pegelow, C.; Kelleher, J.; Presbury, G.; Zarkowsky, H.; Vichinsky, E.; Iyer, R.; Lobel, J.S.; et al. For the Prophylactic Penicillin Study Group. Prophylaxis with oral penicillin in children with sickle cell anemia. A randomized trial. *N. Engl. J. Med.* **1986**, *314*, 1593–1599. [CrossRef] [PubMed]
5. Castilla-Rodríguez, I.; Cela, E.; Vallejo-Torres, L.; Valcárcel-Nazco, C.; Dulín, E.; Espada, M.; Rausell, D.; Mar, J.; Serrano-Aguilar, P. Cost-effectiveness analysis of newborn screening for sickle-cell disease in Spain. *Exp. Opin. Orphan Drugs* **2016**, *4*, 567–575. [CrossRef]
6. Ketelslegers, O.; Eyskens, F.; Boemer, F.; Bours, V.; Minon, J.M.; Gulbis, B. Epidemiological data on sickle cell disease in Belgium. *Belg. J. Hematol.* **2015**, *6*, 135–141.
7. Wolff, F.; Cotton, F.; Gulbis, B. Screening for haemoglobinopathies on cord blood: Laboratory and clinical experience. *J. Med. Screen.* **2012**, *19*, 116–122. [CrossRef] [PubMed]
8. Gulbis, B.; Cotton, F.; Ferster, A.; Ketelslegers, O.; Dresse, M.F.; Rongé-Collard, E.; Minon, J.M.; Lê, P.Q.; Vertongen, F. Neonatal haemoglobinopathy screening in Belgium. *J. Clin. Pathol.* **2009**, *62*, 49–52. [CrossRef] [PubMed]
9. Boemer, F.; Cornet, Y.; Libioulle, C.; Segers, A.; Bours, V.; Schoos, R. 3-Years experience review of neonatal screening for hemoglobin disorders using tandem mass spectrometry. *Clin. Chim. Acta* **2011**, *412*, 1476–1479. [CrossRef] [PubMed]

10. Weatherall, D.J. The inherited diseases of hemoglobin are an emerging global health burden. *Blood* **2010**, *115*, 4331–4436. [CrossRef] [PubMed]
11. Piel, F.B.; Tatem, A.J.; Huang, Z.; Gupta, S.; Williams, T.N.; Weatherall, D.J. Global migration and the changing distribution of sickle haemoglobin: A quantitative study of temporal trends between 1960 and 2000. *Lancet Glob. Health* **2014**, *2*, 80–89. [CrossRef]
12. Migrations en Belgique: Données statistiques. Available online: www.myria.be/files/Migration-rapport-2015-C2.pdf (accessed on 7 October 2018).
13. Vichinsky, E.; Hurst, D.; Earles, A.; Kleman, K.; Lubin, B. Newborn screening for sickle cell disease: Effect on mortality. *Pediatrics* **1988**, *81*, 749–755. [PubMed]
14. King, L.; Fraser, R.; Forbes, M.; Grindley, M.; Ali, S.; Reid, M. Newborn sickle cell disease screening: The Jamaican experience (1995–2006). *J. Med. Screen.* **2007**, *14*, 117–122. [CrossRef] [PubMed]
15. Sabarense, A.P.; Lima, G.O.; Silva, L.M.; Viana, M.B. Survival of children with sickle cell disease in the comprehensive newborn screening programme in Minas Gerais, Brazil. *Paediatr. Int. Child Health* **2015**, *35*, 329–332. [CrossRef] [PubMed]
16. Quinn, C.T.; Rogers, Z.R.; Buchanan, G.R. Survival of children with sickle cell disease. *Blood* **2004**, *103*, 4023–4027. [CrossRef] [PubMed]
17. Quinn, C.T.; Rogers, Z.R.; McCavit, T.L.; Buchanan, G.R. Improved survival of children and adolescents with sickle cell disease. *Blood* **2010**, *115*, 3447–3452. [CrossRef] [PubMed]
18. Lê, P.Q.; Ferster, A.; Dedeken, L.; Vermylen, C.; Vanderfaeillie, A.; Rozen, L.; Heijmans, C.; Huybrechts, S.; Devalck, C.; Efira, A.; et al. Neonatal screening improves sickle cell disease clinical outcome in Belgium. *J. Med. Screen* **2018**, *25*, 57–63. [CrossRef] [PubMed]
19. Couque, N.; Girard, D.; Ducrocq, R.; Boizeau, P.; Haouari, Z.; Misud, F.; Holvoet, L.; Ithier, G.; Belloy, M.; Odièvre, M.H.; et al. Improvement of medical care in a cohort of newborns with sickle-cell disease in North Paris: Impact of national guidelines. *Br. J. Haematol.* **2016**, *173*, 927–937. [CrossRef] [PubMed]

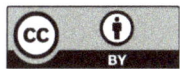 © 2018 by the authors. Licensee MDPI, Basel, Switzerland. This article is an open access article distributed under the terms and conditions of the Creative Commons Attribution (CC BY) license (http://creativecommons.org/licenses/by/4.0/).

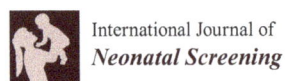

Review

Newborn Screening for SCD in the USA and Canada

Nura El-Haj and Carolyn C. Hoppe *

Department of Hematology-Oncology, UCSF Benioff Children's Hospital Oakland, Oakland, CA 94609, USA; nelhaj@mail.cho.org
* Correspondence: choppe@mail.cho.org; Tel.: +(510)-428-3193

Received: 3 October 2018; Accepted: 20 November 2018; Published: 26 November 2018

Abstract: Sickle cell disease (SCD) encompasses a group of inherited red cell disorders characterized by an abnormal hemoglobin, Hb S. The most common forms of SCD in the United States and Canada are identified through universal newborn screening (NBS) programs. Now carried out in all fifty U.S. states and 8 Canadian provinces, NBS for SCD represents one of the major public health advances in North America. The current status of NBS programs for hemoglobinopathies and the screening techniques employed in many regions worldwide reflect in large part the U.S. and Canadian experiences. Although the structure, screening algorithms and laboratory procedures, as well as reporting and follow up, vary between NBS programs, the overall workflow is similar. The current review summarized the historical background, current approaches, and methods used to screen newborns for SCD in the United States and Canada.

Keywords: hemoglobinopathies; newborn screening; methods; review

1. Introduction

Sickle cell disease (SCD) refers to a clinically heterogeneous group of disorders characterized by a structurally abnormal hemoglobin, hemoglobin S (Hb S), inherited in either a homozygous fashion (Hb SS) or in combination with other Hb variants (e.g., Hb SC, Hb SD, Hb S/O-Arab) or a beta thalassemia mutation (Hb S/beta thalassemia).

Under hypoxic conditions, Hb S polymerizes causing red blood cells to become rigid and deformable [1]. These sickled red blood cells adhere to the vascular endothelium, as well as circulating blood cells, leading to vaso-occlusion and impaired tissue oxygenation [2]. Repeated sickling also damages the red blood cell membrane, resulting in a chronic hemolytic anemia.

Elevated levels of fetal hemoglobin (Hb F) normally present at birth prevent Hb S polymerization and hemolysis and protect affected newborns from complications. As Hb F becomes replaced by Hb S in the first few months of life infants with sickle cell disease (SCD) become at risk for life-threatening complications associated with sickling and hemolysis. These complications, including infection and acute splenic sequestration, are associated with increased morbidity and mortality in the first five years of life [3].

In the USA and Canada, the rationale for newborn hemoglobinopathy screening is based on the benefit provided by penicillin prophylaxis against life-threatening pneumococcal infection in infants with SCD [4]. Since implementation of universal NBS for SCD in the United States, mortality has decreased by 50% in affected children ages 1 to 4 years, and the overall life expectancy has increased from a median of 14.3 years to between 42 and 53 years in males, and between 46 to 58.5 years in females [5]. Additional benefits of NBS include prompt clinical intervention for infection or splenic sequestration episodes, and early education of caretakers about the signs and symptoms of illness in infancy and early childhood [6]. Early parent education on assessment of spleen size reduced mortality due to splenic sequestration by nearly 10-fold in an observational study [7]. Moreover, in a 7-year follow up study, NBS was found to be most effective in reducing mortality when coupled with comprehensive medical care and parent education [5,8].In addition to the public health impact on affected infants, NBS carries the added benefit of identifying at-risk couples, providing the opportunity for genetic counseling regarding options for future pregnancies.

2. Epidemiology

SCD affects over 300,000 newborns per year worldwide [9]. Although hemoglobin disorders are most prevalent in sub-Saharan Africa, throughout Asia, the Middle East, and around the Mediterranean, population migration from these regions has changed the demographic landscape in North America, where the carrier rates for SCD and other hemoglobin disorders have increased in recent years [10]. Contemporary national data regarding the overall prevalence of sickle cell disease in the United States is lacking. However, data derived from the U.S. Census and NBS programs estimates a sickle cell carrier frequency of 8–10% in African-Americans and 0.6% in Hispanics, respectively, and an overall disease prevalence of 100,000 Americans [11].

Using national birth cohort data spanning the 20-year period from 1991–2010, Therrell et al. reported an overall annual birth prevalence of 1:1941 across the USA [12]. Although the absolute number of affected births is lower in Canada, annual birth prevalence rates of SCD in provinces with large multi-ethnic populations, such as Ontario and Quebec, are similar to those in the USA [13]

In Canada, an estimated 3000 to 5000 individuals are living with SCD, the majority of whom reside in Ontario and Quebec. As in the USA, the estimated annual birth incidence of SCD varies geographically with reported estimates of 1:17,721 births in British Columbia, 1:5650 births in Ontario and 1:1852 births in Quebec with the highest rates of 1:2800 births observed in populations of African, Middle Eastern, and Mediterranean descent [14].

3. History of NBS for SCD

The evolution of NBS for SCD, from the initial discovery of a laboratory test to detect sickle hemoglobin to the development of a complex state-based public health program, has been previously described in detail [15]. An overview of the landmark events leading to NBS for SCD is shown in Figure 1. In the USA, population screening for SCD began in the late 1960's in response to mounting political pressure by African American advocacy groups. Only a few states performed testing for SCD in newborns and only on a selective basis.

Evolution of Newborn Screening for Sickle Cell Disease in the USA

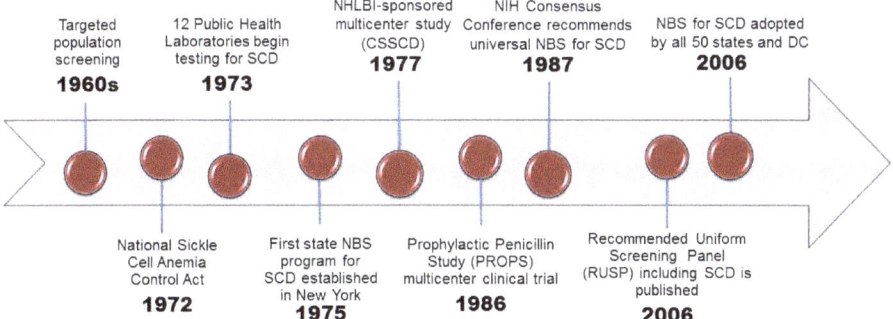

Figure 1. SCD includes Hb SS, Hb S/beta thalassemia and Hb SC genotypes. Abbreviations: ACMG, American College of Medical Genetics; CSSCD, Cooperative Study of Sickle Cell Disease; HHS, Health and Human Services; HRSA, Health Resources and Services Administration; NBS, newborn screening; NHLBI, National Heart, Lung and Blood Institute; NIH, National Institutes of Health; RUSP, Recommended Uniform Screening Panel.

With increasing recognition of SCD as a significant public health issue, Congress passed the National Sickle Cell Anemia Control Act in 1972, which gave authority to establish education, screening, testing, counseling, research, and treatment programs [16]. At the same time, dried blood spots were introduced as an effective method to collect and test blood samples from newborns [17]. By 1973, 12 state public health laboratories had adopted some form of sickle cell screening program and the first statewide NBS program for SCD was established in New York in 1975 [18].

As the first federal program to support a genetic disease, The National Sickle Cell Disease Program funded over 250 general screening programs, 41 sickle cell centers and clinics, as well as 69 research grants and contracts with numerous locally supported screening, education, and counseling clinics [19]. A centralized Hemoglobinopathy Reference Laboratory was also created at the U.S. Centers for Disease Control (CDC) serving as a national resource to assist states in testing for SCD and other hemoglobinopathies, and to provide external proficiency testing and continuing education [20]. After the CDC Hemoglobinopathy Reference Laboratory's closure in 1993, screening and confirmation for all hemoglobin disorders was left to the individual state programs and the proficiency testing program was subsequently transitioned to the Laboratory Quality Assurance Program.

Despite national recognition and federal funding for NBS, states outside of New York, were slow to follow in implementing universal NBS [15,21]. By 1983 only 3 states, New York, Colorado, Texas, had added hemoglobinopathies to the screening panel. The landmark Prophylactic Penicillin Study (PROPS) multicenter clinical trial demonstrating the lifesaving benefit of penicillin prophylaxis against pneumococcal infection in infants and young children with SCD, provided the impetus and justification for universal NBS in the USA [4]. Following publication of this study, the National Institutes of Health convened a consensus conference that resulted in unanimous support for universal NBS for SCD, as mandated by state law [22]. Regionally-centered laboratory services were also recommended in order to improve efficiency and minimize potential errors.

Automated dried blood spot (DBS) punching facilitated expanded screening by significantly reducing the sample preparation time and effort. U.S. and Canadian programs were the first to apply computerized data management to NBS in the 1980s. In 1993, the Agency for Health Care Policy and Research (AHCPR) concluded that NBS for SCD combined with comprehensive health care could significantly reduce infant morbidity and mortality rates, and the agency recommended universal screening rather than targeted screening based on race [23].

By 1999, all but nine states in the USA had implemented universal NBS for SCD. However, there was still no national process to ensure uniformity among states in quality of testing, interpretation of results, or collection of outcome data. In response, the Health Resources and Services Administration commissioned the American College of Medical Genetics to gather expert opinion for a consensus document outlining a core panel of conditions, minimum standards, policies, and procedures for NBS programs nationally [24]. Three SCD genotypes (SS, S/beta thalassemia, and SC) were included in the recommended core panel of state-mandated screening conditions. All other hemoglobinopathies were listed as recommended secondary targets for optional screening. By 2006, all 50 states, the District of Columbia, and many U.S. territories had adopted universal NBS for SCD [15].

Although all NBS programs in the US currently screen for the most common forms of SCD (HbSS, Hb SC, and Hb S/β thalassemia), there are wide variability across states with respect to screening, reporting, and referral of other hemoglobinopathies identified in the course of screening for the core panel conditions. Some states screen for a number of secondary conditions, such as Hb SD, that are concomitantly detected by the screening test methods. A few states have expanded the core screening panel to include clinically relevant non-sickling hemoglobin disorders, such as beta thalassemia and Hb H disease, but most states consider these as secondary screening targets and will refer newborns with a screening test showing a Hb F-only pattern or elevated Bart's hemoglobin for definitive molecular testing [25]. Hemoglobin H disease, an alpha thalassemia disorder prevalent in Southeast Asian, Middle Eastern, and Mediterranean populations, has been given consideration for inclusion as a core condition on the Recommended Uniform Screening Panel (RUSP) RUSP, but lacks sufficient evidence to meet selection criteria [26].

All states require newborn screening, and with the exception of two NBS programs, state statutes that govern screening do not require parental consent. Another 13 states require that parents be informed about NBS prior to testing. All states, except one, allow parents to refuse NBS on religious or personal grounds [27].

Unlike the U.S. where NBS for SCD has been a consideration since 1975, with complete coverage by 2006, screening in Canada was only formalized in one program in 2006, with others slowly coming on board. Targeted screening for SCD began in Quebec in 1988 [13]. The Committee for Development of Newborn Screening for Sickle Cell Disease in Ontario followed in 1989 by launching initiatives and lobbying for universal NBS in Canada. Universal NBS was first implemented in 2006 in Ontario, followed by British Columbia and Yukon in 2009. In 2013, Quebec piloted a universal screening program based on the results from the earlier targeted screening program in Montreal and ultimately implemented a province-wide universal NBS in 2016 [28]. Universal SCD screening is now carried out in 7 Canadian provinces (British Columbia, Ontario, Quebec, New Brunswick, Nova Scotia, Yukon, and Prince Edward Island). Inclusion of SCD on the core NBS panel in Alberta is under consideration pending available funds and service capacity [28].

With no national NBS policy in either the USA or Canada, individual NBS programs screen for a variable number of conditions beyond the recommended core panel, and employ different methods and procedures to carry out screening. Government funding and political support for NBS also vary by region in both countries. Similar to the state governed NBS programs in the USA, universal NBS is under provincial jurisdiction in Canada. Whereas NBS for a recommended core panel of conditions, including SCD, is mandated by individual states in the USA, NBS is considered standard of care in Canada [29]. Moreover, there is no formal province-wide mechanism to document consent, and health care providers are responsible for giving sufficient information to allow parents to make informed decisions, and for documenting parental consent or refusal in the infant's medical record and/or a signed form indicating parent refusal [27].

4. Components of Newborn Screening for SCD

Although logistical aspects, testing methods, and referral policies vary across NBS programs in the United States and Canada, the overarching system for NBS is the same and is comprised of six parts: (1) Education, (2) Screening, (3) Short-Term Follow-Up (STFU), (4) Diagnosis, (5) Management, and (6) Evaluation and Long-Term Follow-Up (LTFU) [30]. NBS programs in both countries follow a similar workflow using newborn DBS specimens, which are tested in specialized screening laboratories and linked to clinical follow-up programs for confirmatory testing and referral to subspecialty comprehensive care [29]. In keeping with national guidelines, state NBS programs in the United States have developed policy and procedure manuals following uniform standards for the performance and documentation of all NBS testing [31].

5. Screening

5.1. Specimen Collection

NBS programs in the United States and Canada have incorporated SCD into the existing laboratory algorithms, and initial screening is now performed in conjunction with testing for other selected congenital disorders. Both countries perform screening using blood spots collected by heel-prick between 24 to 72 h of age, or prior to discharge from the hospital or birthing facility. The timing of collection for repeat blood specimens varies by state. Almost one-third of states require collection of a second sample at age 1–2 weeks [32]. For infants transfused prior to newborn screening, a repeat specimen is recommended between 90 to 120 days after transfusion, unless DNA testing is part of the NBS protocol.

5.2. Specimen Submission

Dried blood spot specimens are sent to a laboratory that is designated by the state or territory within 24–72 h after collection to avoid hemoglobin degradation from prolonged storage and exposure to heat and humidity [33]. Quality checks are performed and the data from the DBS card are entered into a database. Testing is performed within 72 h, typically on the same day the specimen is received in the laboratory.

5.3. Testing Methods

Current methodologies recommended by The Agency for Health Care Policy and Research (AHCPR) for initial and second-tier screening include isoelectric focusing (IEF), high performance liquid chromatography (HPLC), and capillary electrophoresis, which are more sensitive and specific than alkaline and acid gel electrophoresis [34]. Less common screening techniques that are continuing to evolve include tandem mass spectrometry (MS/MS) and various molecular methods [35].

Most NBS programs still use a two-tiered approach, wherein the initial test is followed by a complementary method, such as IEF, HPLC, CE, or dual citrate and cellulose acetate electrophoresis [20]. Alternatively, some NBS laboratories use a modified protocol to improve resolution of the initial test method as the second-tier method. Most NBS laboratories in the US and Canada use HPLC and/or IEF to screen for SCD.

As of 2015, an equal number of NBS laboratories participating in the CDC newborn screen quality assurance proficiency testing program used either HPLC or IEF as the primary screening method [20]. Although HPLC and IEF are highly sensitive and specific, results and interpretation can be confounded by extreme prematurity, previous blood transfusion, or degradation of hemoglobin on the DBS [31].

The increasing availability of automated, reliable, and relatively inexpensive molecular technologies has expanded the use of DNA-based methods for confirmation or definitive diagnosis of NBS results. Molecular techniques can be used either as a second-tier screening method or as a confirmatory test. DNA analysis is performed for second-tier testing in three states (New York, Texas, and Washington). In California, DNA testing on a second specimen is included as part of the screening protocol. In Canada, molecular testing may be requested for NBS results indicating a presumptive β-thalassemia or other genetic variants. Samples are referred to a centralized specialty laboratory for testing at no cost [36].

6. Short Term Follow up

6.1. Primary Screening Results Reporting

As with the provision of NBS laboratory services, follow up and education are also defined by individual NBS programs in both the USA and Canada. Short-term follow up begins with communication of the presumptive positive screening results to the submitting hospital, physician of record, and/or designated NBS follow-up program.

In Canada, all screen-positive test results are reported to the primary care provider, as well as to the provincial Regional Treatment Centers responsible for tracking all presumptive positive cases [36]. The primary care provider (PCP) is given recommendations for the necessary follow up, including initiation of penicillin prophylaxis and is responsible for arranging confirmatory testing on a second liquid blood sample "recall specimen."

A few state NBS programs have incorporated a web-based screening information system allowing follow-up staff at regional coordinating centers and health care providers to directly access the NBS results [37]. This system has been shown to facilitate tracking of positive results and timely enrollment of infants into a comprehensive treatment program.

6.2. Confirmatory Testing

All abnormal or unusual screening results require follow-up of the presumptive screen-positive result through a confirmatory testing protocol to verify the screening result. Policies and practices for confirmatory testing of hemoglobinopathies vary by state. Even in cases where molecular testing on the initial NBS specimen has confirmed the likelihood of a disorder, additional testing is necessary to verify the specimen identification, determine the type of SCD, and to prove or disprove an initial result indicating a presumptive hemoglobinopathy of potential clinical significance. A screening result report of "Other" or "Unknown" hemoglobin variant(s) (often abbreviated as "Hb V") usually indicates the presence of a hemoglobin variant for which the proper comparison to a validated control has not been made. In Canada, confirmatory testing of SCD follows a similar pathway, performed on a liquid blood sample, in contracted reference laboratories, using similar laboratory techniques, either HPLC and/or IEF.

In both the US and Canada, abnormal screening results are reported to a dedicated follow-up agency, sickle cell treatment center or provider to ensure that the newborn and the family have access to appropriate follow-up care. Each US state and Canadian province is responsible for directing its follow-up program state involving NBS program staff, primary care providers, hematologists, and genetic counselors [38]

In the USA, the processes and algorithms for notification and follow-up of newborns with confirmed SCD often place the primary care physician as the initial "medical home," which ideally includes specialists with expertise in SCD, as well as families and community-based organizations working in partnership to obtain the comprehensive services needed. Many states have long-standing contracts with academic SCD and thalassemia centers to provide follow-up services [39]. However, the extent of the comprehensive services provided by the "medical home" is variable and often limited by a lack of resources, competing priorities or incomplete understanding of child health quality measures and care [39].

7. Long-term Follow-up

Long term follow-up is part of the quality assurance component of the NBS system, specifically the evaluation of the effectiveness of the NBS follow-up program in ensuring access to treatment and preventive care throughout the lifespan [40]. In both Canada and the US, treatment and follow-up services are delivered through programs that are either government sponsored, private or public-private collaborations [29]. Currently, all states are required to follow established standards for laboratory practices [41]. All laboratories that perform testing for state NBS programs voluntarily participate in the CDC's Newborn Screening Quality Assurance Program (NSQAP) to verify the accuracy of the screening tests performed.

However, many state programs fall short in tracking the long-term data from comprehensive care centers and specialists, and in evaluating the outcomes. The absence of standard case definitions across states has also been identified as a barrier to aggregate data for comparative analyses. To address this challenge, a HRSA-funded data repository, the Newborn Screening Technical assistance and Evaluation Program (NewSTEPs), was created to facilitate data collection using a uniform nomenclature [42]. These case definitions have been piloted, but not yet validated. State NBS programs are encouraged to utilize the case definitions and to enter case data into the repository [42].

The Health Resources and Services Administration (HRSA)-sponsored Registry and Surveillance System for Hemoglobinopathies (RuSH) is another example of a data resource for evaluating the quality of NBS follow-up by linking multiple data sources across seven states for population-level surveillance of newborns and individuals with SCD [43].

8. Challenges of NBS for SCD

Newborn screening has improved the prognosis for individuals with SCD through early intervention measures, such as penicillin prophylaxis and immunization and early education. However, there remain ongoing challenges with regards to the timely follow-up and implementation of comprehensive care [44]. Wide variation in reporting of screening results by states has led to delays in early intervention [38]. Other states have reported gaps in compliance with early medical intervention, parental education, and the provision of comprehensive health services.

As state NBS programs have different systems for capturing data, the use of different case definitions to evaluate the burden and birth prevalence of SCD has been challenging. Federally-sponsored capacity building for long term follow-up data capture is now a focus across many states, using resources to support coordinated data collection and tracking of cohorts of individuals with SCD to evaluate the long term outcomes [45]. While systems linking state NBS programs using common data definitions are in development, there is currently no mechanism linking NBS systems with clinical data systems, nor is there a standardized approach to assess the impact of NBS on health outcomes in children.

Patient registries using medical record linkage with NBS programs are being explored to facilitate the transfer and exchange of information between the NBS program and clinical providers [46]. Health information technology (e.g., electronic medical record exchanges and interoperability standards) provides a tool for consistent data collection, current care practices, and identifying gaps. The costs associated with building this capacity for long term follow-up remains a major challenge. Moreover, the decline in reimbursement for services from public insurance programs has further limited the ability to provide adequate clinical care and education to affected patients [23].

Only a few NBS programs have established activities focused on policy development and system change [47]. Despite the recently published NHLBI evidence-based clinical standards of care for SCD, the available preventative and therapeutic interventions are not reaching the affected individuals [48]. A framework for widespread application of the NHLBI guidelines, using implementation science methods, has been proposed to close the "quality gap" [47].

9. Conclusion

The history of NBS for SCD in the USA and Canada spans many years beginning with the recognition of SCD as a significant public health issue, and the identification of hemoglobinopathies from the same dried blood spot used to screen for other congenital disorders. Many of the screening tests that have become part of routine screening worldwide were initially developed in the U.S. and Canadian laboratories, including hemoglobinopathy testing. In both countries, the components of NBS include a screening process incorporating specimen collection, submission, and a two-tiered testing approach using complementary methods to identify a hemoglobinopathy. However, NBS programs in both countries use different methods of testing and reporting results to public health programs, hospitals, and individual providers, with wide variation in the content and format. Although the implementation of NBS for SCD has led to improved outcomes in children, few studies have evaluated the long-term health outcomes in the growing population of adults with SCD. Efforts to standardize nomenclature and collection of outcomes data through the development of linked registries are a first step in achieving the long-term follow-up goal to ensure appropriate delivery of health care to individuals with SCD identified by the NBS.

Author Contributions: For research articles with several authors, a short paragraph specifying their individual contributions must be provided. The following statements should be used "Conceptualization, N.E.-H. and C.C.H.; Data Curation, N.E.-H.; Writing-Original Draft Preparation, N.E.-H.; Writing-Review & Editing, N.E.-H. and C.C.H.; Supervision, C.C.H.

Funding: This research received no external funding.

Conflicts of Interest: The authors declare no conflict of interest.

References

1. Brittenham, G.M.; Schechter, A.N.; Noguchi, C.T. Hemoglobin S polymerization: Primary determinant of the hemolytic and clinical severity of the sickling syndromes. *Blood* **1985**, *65*, 183–189. [PubMed]
2. Frenette, P.S. Sickle cell vaso-occlusion: Multistep and multicellular paradigm. *Curr. Opin. Hematol.* **2002**, *9*, 101–106. [CrossRef] [PubMed]
3. Gill, F.M.; Sleeper, L.A.; Weiner, S.J.; Brown, A.K.; Bellevue, R.; Grover, R.; Pegelow, C.H.; Vichinsky, E. Clinical events in the first decade in a cohort of infants with sickle cell disease. Cooperative Study of Sickle Cell Disease. *Blood* **1995**, *86*, 776–783. [PubMed]
4. Gaston, M.H.; Verter, J.I.; Woods, G.; Pegelow, C.; Kelleher, J.; Presbury, G.; Zarkowsky, H.; Vichinsky, E.; Iyer, R.; Lobel, J.S.; et al. Prophylaxis with oral penicillin in children with sickle cell anemia. A randomized trial. *N. Engl. J. Med.* **1986**, *314*, 1593–1599. [CrossRef] [PubMed]
5. Vichinsky, E.; Hurst, D.; Earles, A.; Kleman, K.; Lubin, B. Newborn screening for sickle cell disease: Effect on mortality. *Pediatrics* **1988**, *81*, 749–755. [PubMed]
6. Frempong, T.; Pearson, H.A. Newborn screening coupled with comprehensive follow-up reduced early mortality of sickle cell disease in Connecticut. *Connect. Med.* **2007**, *71*, 9–12.
7. Emond, A.M.; Collis, R.; Darvill, D.; Higgs, D.R.; Maude, G.H.; Serjeant, G.R. Acute splenic sequestration in homozygous sickle cell disease: Natural history and management. *J. Pediatr.* **1985**, *107*, 201–206. [CrossRef]
8. Vichinsky, E.P. Comprehensive care in sickle cell disease: Its impact on morbidity and mortality. *Semin. Hematol.* **1991**, *28*, 220–226. [PubMed]
9. Piel, F.B. The Present and future global burden of the inherited disorders of hemoglobin. *Hematol. Oncol. Clin. North. Am.* **2016**, *30*, 327–341. [CrossRef] [PubMed]
10. Piel, F.B.; Tatem, A.J.; Huang, Z.; Gupta, S.; Williams, T.N.; Weatherall, D.J. Global migration and the changing distribution of sickle haemoglobin: A quantitative study of temporal trends between 1960 and 2000. *Lancet Glob. Health* **2014**, *2*, e80–e89. [CrossRef]
11. Hassell, K.L. Population estimates of sickle cell disease in the U.S. *Am. J. Prev. Med.* **2010**, *38* (Suppl. 4), S512–S521. [CrossRef] [PubMed]
12. Therrell, B.L., Jr.; Lloyd-Puryear, M.A.; Eckman, J.R.; Mann, M.Y. Newborn screening for sickle cell diseases in the United States: A review of data spanning 2 decades. *Semin. Perinatol.* **2015**, *39*, 238–251. [CrossRef] [PubMed]
13. Robitaille, N.; Delvin, E.E.; Hume, H.A. Newborn screening for sickle cell disease: A 1988-2003 Quebec experience. *Paediatr. Child Health* **2006**, *11*, 223–227. [CrossRef] [PubMed]
14. Davies, C.; Potter, B.K.; Khangura, M.; Hawken, S.; Hawken, J. Epidemiology and health system impact of hemoglobinopathy: Results from Newborn Screening Ontario. 2015 Canadian Newborn and Child Screening Symposium, Ottawa, ON, Canada, 30 April–1 May 2015.
15. Benson, J.M.; Therrell, B.L., Jr. History and current status of newborn screening for hemoglobinopathies. *Semin. Perinatol.* **2010**, *34*, 134–144. [CrossRef] [PubMed]
16. *National Sickle Cell Anemia Control Act*; US Congress: Washington, DC, USA, 1972; Volume 86, p. 136.
17. Garrick, M.D.; Dembure, P.; Guthrie, R. Sickle-cell anemia and other hemoglobinopathies. Procedures and strategy for screening employing spots of blood on filter paper as specimens. *N. Engl. J. Med.* **1973**, *288*, 1265–1268. [CrossRef] [PubMed]
18. Grover, R.; Shahidi, S.; Fisher, B.; Goldberg, D.; Wethers, D. Current sickle cell screening program for newborns in New York City, 1979–1980. *Am. J. Public Health* **1983**, *73*, 249–252. [CrossRef] [PubMed]
19. Schmidt, R.M. Hemoglobinopathy screening: Approaches to diagnosis, education and counseling. *Am. J. Public Health* **1974**, *64*, 799–804. [CrossRef] [PubMed]
20. Laboratories, A.O.P.H. *Hemoglobinopathies: Current Practices for Screening, Confirmation and Follow up*; Centers for Disease Control: Atlanta, GA, USA, 2015.
21. Selekman, J. Update: New guidelines for the treatment of infants with sickle cell disease. Agency for Health Care Policy and Research. *Pediatr. Nurs.* **1993**, *19*, 600–605. [PubMed]
22. Consensus conference. Newborn screening for sickle cell disease and other hemoglobinopathies. *JAMA* **1987**, *258*, 1205–1209. [CrossRef]
23. Smith, J.A.; Kinney, T.R. Sickle cell disease: Screening and management in newborns and infants. Agency for Health Care Policy and Research. *Am. Fam. Phys.* **1993**, *48*, 95–102.

24. Newborn screening: Toward a uniform screening panel and system-executive summary. *Pediatrics* **2006**, *117*, S296–S307. [CrossRef] [PubMed]
25. Calonge, N.; Green, N.S.; Rinaldo, P.; Lloyd-Puryear, M.; Dougherty, D.; Boyle, C.; Watson, M.; Trotter, T.; Terry, S.F.; Howell, R.R.; et al. Committee report: Method for evaluating conditions nominated for population-based screening of newborns and children. *Genet. Med.* **2010**, *12*, 153–159. [CrossRef] [PubMed]
26. Knapp, A.A.; Metterville, D.R.; Kemper, A.R.; Perrin, J.M. *Newborn Screening for Hemoglobin H Disease: A Summary of the Evidence and Advisory Committee Decision*; Health Resources and Services Administration: Rockville, MD, USA, 2010.
27. Hiller, E.H.; Landenburger, G.; Natowicz, M.R. Public participation in medical policy-making and the status of consumer autonomy: The example of newborn-screening programs in the United States. *Am. J. Public Health* **1997**, *87*, 1280–1288. [CrossRef] [PubMed]
28. *Newborn Blood Spot Screening for Galactosemia, Tyrosinemia Type 1, Homocystinuria, Sickle Cell Anemia, Sickle Cell/Beta-Thallassemia, Sickle Cell/Hemoglobin C Disease and Severe Combined Immunodeficiency: Costs and Cost Analysis*; 2016-03; Institute of Health Economics: Edmonton, AB, Canada, 2016.
29. Therrell, B.L.; Adams, J. Newborn screening in North America. *J. Inherit. Metab. Dis.* **2007**, *30*, 447–465. [CrossRef] [PubMed]
30. Therrell, B.L.; Hannon, W.H. National evaluation of US newborn screening system components. *Ment. Retard. Dev. Disabil. Res. Rev.* **2006**, *12*, 236–245. [CrossRef] [PubMed]
31. Campbell, M.; Henthorn, J.S.; Davies, S.C. Evaluation of cation-exchange HPLC compared with isoelectric focusing for neonatal hemoglobinopathy screening. *Clin. Chem.* **1999**, *45*, 969–975. [PubMed]
32. CLSI Document NBS01-A6. *Blood Collection on Filter Paper for Newborn Screening Programs*, 6th ed.; Approved Standard; CLSI: Wayne, PA, USA, 2013.
33. Adam, B.W.; Haynes, C.A.; Chafin, D.L.; De Jesus, V.R. Stabilities of intact hemoglobin molecules and hemoglobin peptides in dried blood samples. *Clin. Chim. Acta* **2014**, *429*, 59–60. [CrossRef] [PubMed]
34. Huisman, T.H. Separation of hemoglobins and hemoglobin chains by high-performance liquid chromatography. *J. Chromatogr.* **1987**, *418*, 277–304. [CrossRef]
35. Boemer, F.; Ketelslegers, O.; Minon, J.M.; Bours, V.; Schoos, R. Newborn screening for sickle cell disease using tandem mass spectrometry. *Clin. Chem.* **2008**, *54*, 2036–2041. [CrossRef] [PubMed]
36. Newborn Screening Ontario. Regional Treatment Centres. Available online: https://www.newbornscreening.on.ca/en/health-care-providers/regional-treatment-centres (accessed on 28 September 2018).
37. Feuchtbaum, L.; Dowray, S.; Lorey, F. The context and approach for the California newborn screening short- and long-term follow-up data system: Preliminary findings. *Genet. Med.* **2010**, *12* (Suppl. 12), S242–S250. [CrossRef]
38. Kavanagh, P.L.; Wang, C.J.; Therrell, B.L.; Sprinz, P.G.; Bauchner, H. Communication of positive newborn screening results for sickle cell disease and sickle cell trait: Variation across states. *Am. J. Med. Genet. Part C Semin. Med. Genet.* **2008**, *148C*, 15–22. [CrossRef] [PubMed]
39. Hinton, C.F.; Feuchtbaum, L.; Kus, C.A.; Kemper, A.R.; Berry, S.A.; Levy-Fisch, J.; Luedtke, J.; Kaye, C.; Boyle, C.A. What questions should newborn screening long-term follow-up be able to answer? A statement of the US Secretary for Health and Human Services' Advisory Committee on Heritable Disorders in Newborns and Children. *Genet. Med.* **2011**, *13*, 861–865. [CrossRef] [PubMed]
40. Kemper, A.R.; Boyle, C.A.; Aceves, J.; Dougherty, D.; Figge, J.; Fisch, J.L.; Hinman, A.R.; Greene, C.L.; Kus, C.A.; Miller, J.; et al. Long-term follow-up after diagnosis resulting from newborn screening: Statement of the US Secretary of Health and Human Services' Advisory Committee on Heritable Disorders and Genetic Diseases in Newborns and Children. *Genet. Med. Off. J. Am. Coll. Med. Genet.* **2008**, *10*, 259–261. [CrossRef] [PubMed]
41. Centers for Disease. Prevention, Good laboratory practices for biochemical genetic testing and newborn screening for inherited metabolic disorders. *MMWR. Recomm. Rep. Morb. Mortal. Wkly. Rep. Recomm. Rep.* **2012**, *61*, 1–44.
42. Sontag, M.K.; Sarkar, D.; Comeau, A.M.; Hassell, K.; Botto, L.D.; Parad, R.; Rose, S.R.; Wintergerst, K.A.; Smith-Whitley, K.; Singh, S.; et al. Case definitions for conditions identified by newborn screening public health surveillance. *Int. J. Neonatal Screen.* **2018**, *4*, 16. [CrossRef] [PubMed]

43. Paulukonis, S.T.; Harris, W.T.; Coates, T.D.; Neumayr, L.; Treadwell, M.; Vichinsky, E.; Feuchtbaum, L.B. Population based surveillance in sickle cell disease: Methods, findings and implications from the California registry and surveillance system in hemoglobinopathies project (RuSH). *Pediatr. Blood Cancer* **2014**, *61*, 2271–2276. [CrossRef] [PubMed]
44. Sox, H.C. Resolving the tension between population health and individual health care. *JAMA* **2013**, *310*, 1933–1934. [CrossRef] [PubMed]
45. Wharton, M.; Chorba, T.L.; Vogt, R.L.; Morse, D.L.; Buehler, J.W. *Case Definitions for Public Health Surveillance*; U.S. Department of Health and Human Services: Atlanta, GA, USA, 1990; pp. 1–43.
46. Wang, Y.; Caggana, M.; Sango-Jordan, M.; Sun, M.; Druschel, C.M. Long-term follow-up of children with confirmed newborn screening disorders using record linkage. *Genet. Med.* **2011**, *13*, 881–886. [CrossRef] [PubMed]
47. DiMartino, L.D.; Baumann, A.A.; Hsu, L.L.; Kanter, J.; Gordeuk, V.R.; Glassberg, J.; Treadwell, M.J.; Melvin, C.L.; Telfair, J.; Klesges, L.M.; et al. The sickle cell disease implementation consortium: Translating evidence-based guidelines into practice for sickle cell disease. *Am. J. Hematol.* **2018**. [CrossRef] [PubMed]
48. Hassell, T.; Hennis, A. Chronic Disease Challenges in the Caribbean. *Glob. Heart* **2016**, *11*, 437–438. [CrossRef] [PubMed]

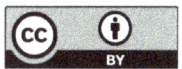

© 2018 by the authors. Licensee MDPI, Basel, Switzerland. This article is an open access article distributed under the terms and conditions of the Creative Commons Attribution (CC BY) license (http://creativecommons.org/licenses/by/4.0/).

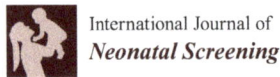

Article

Newborn Screening for Sickle Cell Disease in the Caribbean: An Update of the Present Situation and of the Disease Prevalence

Jennifer Knight-Madden [1], Ketty Lee [2], Gisèle Elana [3], Narcisse Elenga [4], Beatriz Marcheco-Teruel [5], Ngozi Keshi [6], Maryse Etienne-Julan [7], Lesley King [1], Monika Asnani [1], Marc Romana [8,9,†] and Marie-Dominique Hardy-Dessources [8,9,10,*,†] on behalf of the CAREST Network

[1] Caribbean Institute for Health Research—Sickle Cell Unit, The University of the West Indies, Mona, Kingston 7, Jamaica; jennifer.knightmadden@uwimona.edu.jm (J.K.-M.); lesley.king@uwimona.edu.jm (L.K.); monika.parshadasnani@uwimona.edu.jm (M.A.)
[2] Laboratory of Molecular Genetics, Academic Hospital of Guadeloupe, 97159 Pointe-à-Pitre, Guadeloupe; ketty.lee@chu-guadeloupe.fr
[3] Referral Center for Sickle Cell Disease, Department of Pediatrics, Academic Hospital of Martinique, 97261 Fort de France, Martinique, France; gisele.elana@chu-martinique.fr
[4] Referral Center for Sickle Cell Disease, Department of Pediatric Medicine and Surgery, Andrée Rosemon General Hospital, 97306 Cayenne, French Guiana, France; narcisse.elenga@ch-cayenne.fr
[5] National Center of Medical Genetics, 11300 La Habana, Cuba; beatriz@infomed.sld.cu
[6] Paediatric Department, Scarborough General Hospital, 00000 Scarborough, Tobago; nzigokeshi@yahoo.com
[7] Referral Center for Sickle Cell Disease, Sickle Cell Unit, Academic Hospital of Guadeloupe, 97159 Pointe-à-Pitre, Guadeloupe, France; maryse.etienne-julan@chu-guadeloupe.fr
[8] UMR Inserm 1134 Biologie Intégrée du Globule Rouge, Inserm/Université Paris Diderot—Université Sorbonne Paris Cité/INTS/Université des Antilles, Hôpital Ricou, Academic Hospital of Guadeloupe, 97159 Pointe-à-Pitre, Guadeloupe; marc.romana@inserm.fr
[9] Laboratoire d'Excellence du Globule Rouge (Labex GR-Ex), PRES Sorbonne, 75015 Paris, France
[10] CAribbean Network of REsearchers on Sickle Cell Disease and Thalassemia, UMR Inserm 1134, Hôpital Ricou, Academic Hospital of Guadeloupe, 97159 Pointe-à-Pitre, Guadeloupe
* Correspondence: marie-dominique.hardy-dessources@inserm.fr; Tel.: (+590)-590-83-48-99
† These authors contributed equally to this work.

Received: 13 November 2018; Accepted: 1 January 2019; Published: 8 January 2019

Abstract: The region surrounding the Caribbean Sea is predominantly composed of island nations for its Eastern part and the American continental coast on its Western part. A large proportion of the population, particularly in the Caribbean islands, traces its ancestry to Africa as a consequence of the Atlantic slave trade during the XVI–XVIII centuries. As a result, sickle cell disease has been largely introduced in the region. Some Caribbean countries and/or territories, such as Jamaica and the French territories, initiated newborn screening (NBS) programs for sickle cell disease more than 20 years ago. They have demonstrated the major beneficial impact on mortality and morbidity resulting from early childhood care. However, similar programs have not been implemented in much of the region. This paper presents an update of the existing NBS programs and the prevalence of sickle cell disease in the Caribbean. It demonstrates the impact of the Caribbean Network of Researchers on Sickle Cell Disease and Thalassemia (CAREST) on the extension of these programs. The presented data illustrate the importance of advocacy in convincing policy makers of the feasibility and benefit of NBS for sickle cell disease when coupled to early care.

Keywords: sickle cell disease; newborn screening; Caribbean

1. Introduction

The Caribbean is defined as the geographical region including the Caribbean Sea, more than 700 islands, and the surrounding coasts. The region is located southeast of the Gulf of Mexico and the North American mainland, East of Central America, and North of South America. A wider definition includes Belize, the Caribbean region of Colombia, the Yucatán Peninsula, and the Guyanas (Guyana, Suriname, French Guiana, the Guyana region in Venezuela, and the state of Amapà in Brazil); these areas have political and cultural ties to the region. The Caribbean islands are organized into 13 sovereign states and 17 overseas territories/departments and dependencies, with 43 million inhabitants and at least five official spoken languages.

The Caribbean countries and territories share some common historical features. Less than two centuries after the arrival of Christopher Columbus in the New World, these territories were all under the rules of the European colonial powers (France, United Kingdom, Spain, Portugal, The Netherlands, and Denmark). The introduction of new crops which needed intensive work, such as tobacco, cotton, and sugarcane, led to the development of the transatlantic slave trade. More than 12 million Africans were deported to the New World [1]. One of the consequences of this massive forced migration was the introduction of sickle cell disease (SCD) into the New World. The migration of Indians as indentured laborers when slavery was abolished led to the introduction of the Arabo-Indian haplotype of the β^S gene and thalassemia alleles.

The Caribbean occupies a unique position in the history of SCD in the modern era. Indeed, the first case ever described in the Western medical literature by Herricks in 1910 was that of a young fellow from Grenada studying dentistry in Chicago (USA) [2]. Additionally, the benefits of newborn screening (NBS) for SCD as a public health tool, including evidence of both the feasibility of the test and its major impact on mortality and morbidity, were first demonstrated in Jamaica [3]. Available data also suggest that the prevalence of SCD in the Caribbean Region is second only to Sub-Saharan Africa [4].

However, prior to 2006, accurate SCD prevalence and epidemiological data were available for only a limited number of these countries and territories. These data were provided from NBS programs implemented in Jamaica [5] and in the French territories [6], as well as from a prenatal diagnosis program in Cuba [7,8]. Collaboration between medical and scientific Caribbean teams began to increase in 2006, leading to the founding in 2011 of the Caribbean Network of Researchers on Sickle Cell Disease and Thalassemia (CAREST) as a not-for-profit organization [9]. Promotion of NBS for the hemoglobinopathies and assistance for the establishment of sickle cell centers were the primary goals of CAREST. CAREST has worked with all regional stakeholders with common goals, including the SickKids Caribbean Initiative. It has included outreach initiatives to clinicians and policy makers to share regional data regarding the status of SCD NBS and the implications for their own countries. As a result, we present an SCD NBS program initiated in Tobago since 2008 and pilot NBS programs conducted in Grenada and Saint Lucia in 2014–2015 and 2015–2017, respectively.

Beyond the presentation and discussion on the experience of CAREST in establishing NBS programs, we also present an update on the prevalence of SCD in the Caribbean.

2. Materials and Methods

2.1. Neonatal Screening for Sickle Cell Disease

Blood samples obtained neonatally are collected on Guthrie cards. As shown in Table 1, cord blood samples are collected in Martinique, Jamaica, and St Lucia, whereas in Guadeloupe, Tobago, Grenada, and French Guiana, heel prick samples are obtained. Heel prick samples were also collected for the Saint Lucia's pilot NBS project funded by the SickKids Caribbean Initiative (2015–2017) and these samples were sent and processed in Jamaica. This project sought to test the feasibility of replacing cord blood sampling and hemoglobin electrophoresis which had been in place since 1992, by heel prick sampling and high-performance liquid chromatography (HPLC); during the pilot, both systems ran concomitantly. Blood samples from Tobago and Grenada are sent by post-mail and analyzed in Guadeloupe (Table 1).

Table 1. Neonatal screening process.

Site	Sample	Screening Center	First Test	Confirmation Test
Guadeloupe Tobago Grenada	Heel prick/Guthrie cards	Guadeloupe	HPLC	IEF
Martinique	Cord blood/Guthrie cards	Martinique	IEF	HPLC
French Guiana	Heel prick/Guthrie cards	France (Lille)	CE	HPLC
Jamaica 1995–2015 Jamaica 2015–2018	Cord blood/Guthrie cards	Jamaica	Citrate agar HPLC	Cellulose acetate IEF
Saint Lucia 1992–2018 [†] Saint Lucia 2015–2017 [††]	Cord blood/Guthrie cards Heel prick/Guthrie cards	Saint-Lucia Jamaica	Citrate agar HPLC	Cellulose acetate IEF

[†] From Alexander et al. [10]; [††] From pilot (results not previously published). HPLC: high-performance liquid chromatography; IEF: isoelectric focusing; CE: capillary electrophoresis.

As indicated in Table 1, the samples are primarily tested in reference laboratories based in Guadeloupe (University Hospital of Guadeloupe), Martinique (University Hospital of Martinique), and Jamaica (Sickle Cell Unit, Caribbean Institute for Health Research, Kingston and Southern Regional Health Authority, Manchester). French Guiana specimens are sent to a reference laboratory based in mainland France (regional center for metabolic disease screening, Lille). Saint Lucian cord blood samples, except for those obtained during the pilot study, are tested locally.

NBS itself now primarily uses three laboratory-based methodologies for detecting Hb variants: isoelectric focusing (IEF), capillary electrophoresis (CE), and high-performance liquid chromatography (HPLC), one is used as the first-line screening method and a second as a confirmatory test. In Saint Lucia, however, hemoglobin cellulose acetate and citrate agar electrophoresis are used locally for cord blood samples. In Guadeloupe, DNA analysis is also secondarily performed as a confirmatory diagnosis of a new sample (peripheral blood on EDTA as anticoagulant) in the following cases: FS phenotype when the two parents cannot be tested in order to distinguish SS, S/beta-thalassemia, or S/HPFH; and the FSX or FCX phenotype in order to formally identify the abnormal hemoglobin (HbX), as well as for ambiguous primary screening results [11,12].

2.2. Prenatal Screening for SCD

In Cuba, the screening for SCD is a prenatal diagnosis based on fetal DNA analysis. This procedure has been established since 1982 for mothers at risk and the screening program is performed on pregnant women at the provincial centers of genetics located all over the country [7,8].

2.3. Initiation of Early Childhood Care for SCD

Children confirmed to have a diagnosis of SCD are enrolled in the different sickle cell centers or clinical structures as soon as possible to initiate clinical management and to provide information to the parents. To shorten delays and promote early medical management of the newly identified SCD children from Tobago, the results are sent by e-mail from the laboratory in Guadeloupe to the appropriate health care provider using secure file transfer systems. Similar communication procedures were also used during the pilot projects in Grenada and Saint Lucia.

2.4. Data Analysis

Allele frequencies were estimated by gene-counting and the prevalence of SCD was calculated from the newborn screening results.

3. Results

Table 2 summarizes the main results of the hemoglobinopathy NBS programs performed in the French territories [6], Jamaica [5], Grenada [13], Tobago [9], and Saint Lucia [10].

Table 2. Results from the newborn screening programs in the Caribbean.

Site	Period	Number of Samples Screened	FAS	FAC	FS	FSC	FC	Other
Jamaica	1995–2006 *	150,803	14,688 9.74% 9.59–9.89%	5420 3.59% 3.50–3.69%	557 0.37% 0.34–0.40%	332 0.22% 0.20–0.25%	115 0.08 0.06–0.09%	972 0.64% 0.61–0.69%
	2016–2017	40,444	4020 9.94% 9.65–10.24	1481 3.66% 3.48–3.85	165 0.41% 0.35–0.47	95 0.23% 0.19–0.29	35 0.09% 0.06–0.12	63 0.16% 0.12–0.20
Guadeloupe	1984–2010	178,428	14,126 7.92% 7.79–8.04%	4375 2.45% 2.38–2.52%	310 0.17% 0.16–0.19%	231 0.13% 0.11–0.15%	39 0.02 0.02–0.03%	248 0.14 0.12–0.16%
Martinique	2009–2015 **	30,171	2134 7.07% 6.79–7.37%	910 3.02% 2.83–3.22%	44 0.15% 0.11–0.20%	29 0.10% 0.07–0.14%	11 0.04% 0.02–0.07%	88 0.29% 0.29–0.36%
French Guiana	1992–2013	115,200	8824 7.66% 7.51–7.81%	2797 2.43% 2.34–2.52%	293 0.25% 0.23–0.29%	186 0.16% 0.14–0.19%	NA	NA
Grenada	2014–2015	1914	183 (9.56%) 8.32–10.96%	63 3.29% 2.58–4.19%	10 0.52% 0.28–0.96%	2 0.10% 0.03–0.38%	1 0.05% 0.01–0.3%	2 0.10% 0.03–0.38%
Tobago	2008–2017	7389	689 9.32% 8.68–10.01%	285 3.86% 3.44–4.32%	28 0.38% 0.26–0.55%	14 0.19% 0.11–0.32%	5 0.07% 0.03–0.16%	21 0.28% 0.19–0.43%
St Lucia	1992–2010 †	36,253	3146 8.68% 8.39–8.97%	NA	180 0.50% 0.43–0.57%	59 0.16% 0.13–0.21%	NA	NA
	2015–2017 ††	2023	238 11.76% 10.43–13.24%	42 2.08% 1.54–2.79%	3 0.15% 0.05–0.44%	5 0.25% 0.11–0.58%	2 0.10% 0.04–3.6%	NA

Number of samples screened with the FAS, FAC, FS, and FSC phenotypes are indicated (first line), as well as the prevalence (%) and (95% confidence interval). Other: samples presenting with an abnormal hemoglobin other than HbS or HbC; NA: Not available; * samples collected under the South–East Regional Jamaican Health Authorities only and tested at the Sickle Cell Unit, Caribbean Institute for Health Research (from King et al. [5]); ** universal screening was initiated in Martinique in 1986 in two different laboratories and in 2009, it was centralized in one single center; reliable data are only available from 2009 onwards; † from Alexander et al. [10]; †† From pilot (results not previously published).

The current coverage of the NBS programs is as follows: Guadeloupe (>98%), Martinique (>99%), Jamaica (>98%), and Tobago (96%). The coverage of the two pilot NBSs in Grenada and Saint Lucia were 79% and 45% respectively. In Cuba, since the beginning of the program until December 2016, 7659 couples at risk have been identified.

The highest frequency of sickle cell trait carriers is observed in Jamaica (9.74–9.94%), Grenada (9.56%), and Tobago (9.32%). In Jamaica, less samples presenting abnormal hemoglobin other than HbS or HbC have been observed during the 2016–2017 period (0.16%) than during the previous screening period (0.64%), probably due to an optimization of the Hb variant detection.

The low screening coverage rate (45%) in Saint-Lucia during the period 2015–2017 could explain the differences in the frequency of phenotypes observed compared to the 1992–2010 period.

Table 3 summarizes the currently available data on β^S and β^C allele frequencies, carrier prevalence, and SCD prevalence in the Caribbean area.

Table 3. SCD birth prevalence in the Caribbean countries and territories.

(A) Neonatal Screening					
Country/Territory	Screening Method	Carrier Prevalence (Hb S and Hb C Trait)	Gene Frequencies	β^S/β^C Ratio	SCD Prevalence
Jamaica	Specific locations (1995–2006) [6]	15%	β^S: 0.055–β^C: 0.019	2.89	0.53%–1/188
	Univ screen (2016–2017)	13.6%	β^S: 0.055–β^C: 0.020	2.75	0.65%–1/153
Guadeloupe	Univ screen	10.5%	β^S: 0.042–β^C: 0.013	3.23	0.33%–1/304
Martinique	Univ screen	10%	β^S: 0.040–β^C: 0.012	3.33	0.31%–1/322
French Guiana	Univ screen	10%	β^S: 0.039–β^C: 0.012	3.25	0.42%–1/235
Tobago	Univ screen	13.2%	β^S: 0.051–β^C: 0.021	2.43	0.57%–1/176
Grenada [7]	Univ screen	12.85%	β^S: 0.054–β^C: 0.018	3.00	0.63%–1/160
Saint Lucia	Univ screen	13.8%	β^S: 0.062–β^C: 0.013	4.77	0.39%–1/253
Haiti [9]	Pilot screen	13.46%	β^S: 0.059–β^C: 0.013	4.54	0.58%–1/173
Saint Vincent & Grenadines [10]	Pilot screen	15.27%	β^S: 0.065–β^C: 0.016	4.06	0.26%–1/382
(B) Prenatal Diagnosis					
Country/Territory	Screening Method	Carrier Prevalence (Hb S and Hb C Trait)	Gene Frequencies	β^S/β^C Ratio	SCD Prevalence
Cuba	Prenatal diagnosis	3.1%	β^S: 0.011–β^C: 0.0036 [a]	3.06	
			β^S: 0.053–β^C: 0.006 [b]	8.83	0.02%–1/5000

Univ screen: universal screening; [a]: Figures for the Western side of Cuba (not including for Havana); [b]: figures for the Southeastern side of Cuba.

Several abnormal genotypes, some of which include hemoglobin variants leading to sickle cell disease when associated with the β^S allele, have also been identified during the course of these NBS programs. Indeed, the second most frequent sickle cell genotype encountered in these populations was the genotype SC, with some differences in the β^S/β^C ratio detected, and the highest was observed in Saint-Lucia and the lowest in Tobago, as indicated in Table 3. The others correspond to S/β-thalassemia compound heterozygosity (including S/E and S/Lepore) and also S/D^{Punjab} [3,6].

Once infants are screened, confirmation and referral for care are ensued. In French speaking territories and in Jamaica, care is provided according to the guidelines of the French Health Authority [14] and the Sickle Cell Unit [15], respectively. The Sickle Cell Unit Clinical Care Guidelines are currently in use in several other Anglophone countries, including Trinidad and Tobago, Saint-Lucia, the Bahamas, and Barbados. The focus is on pneumococcal prevention and general health maintenance (parents' education, counselling) prior to the onset of complications. In Martinique, Guadeloupe, French Guiana, and Jamaica, most of the SCD children identified by the NBS program are followed by Sickle cell centers before the age of three months [5,6]. In Saint-Lucia and Tobago, babies identified are followed up in pediatric outpatient clinics. In Cuba, guidelines for management and treatment have also been developed [8].

4. Discussion

Given the SCD prevalence and the demonstration of the benefit of the NBS program, one might have expected that SCD NBS would be entrenched across the Region. This is clearly not the case and our data suggest several factors which may be at play, with the availability of resources being a major issue [5,6,9].

Caribbean territories which are part of larger states which mandate SCD NBS as part of a larger universal NBS program, have long and well-established programs. These may be the best funded programs in the Region. In the three French territories, Guadeloupe, Martinique, and French Guiana, the cost of the test is borne by the French government. In territories of the United States of America, screening started in Puerto Rico in 1977 and the US Virgin Islands in 1987 [16]. The test mandated by law covers 99% of births, but the hospitals include a charge to the patient for the NBS panel (http://bft.stage.bbox.ly/newborn-screening/states/puerto-rico). Overseas British territories have separate health systems and SCD NBS is not uniformly offered.

Among the independent nations, Cuba has an integrated public health program and SCD prenatal testing for couples at risk and carrier women was mandated by law in 1983 [7,8]. This program seeks to actively prevent the births of children with SCD, and is perhaps the most active in promoting the termination of pregnancies; since termination of pregnancy was requested by 76.5% of at-risk couples.

In the other independent Caribbean nations, screening varies based on factors such as historical context, current champions, and public health commitment. Jamaica has a unique historical context as the site of the Jamaica Sickle Cell Cohort Study. Nevertheless, after the completion of recruitment for the cohort study in 1981, SCD NBS ceased until 1995, when, through the advocacy of the Sickle Cell Support Club of Jamaica (now the Sickle Cell Support Foundation), it was restarted. For a decade, it was limited to three hospitals in the South East Regional Health Authority, providing screening for approximately 43% of all national births. The coverage gradually increased from 2008 to 2015 when essentially universal coverage was achieved. While testing was mandated in the National Strategic Plan for the Prevention and Control of Non-communicable Disease in Jamaica 2012–2018, there is no legislative mandate and the integration of the program into the fabric of the public health system remains incomplete. Thus, the sustainability of the program depends on the support of incumbent policy makers.

The Saint Lucia Sickle Cell Association (SSCA), a local non-governmental organization, has been strong for many years. It was influential in the introduction of universal SCD NBS in 1992 and its integration into the Ministry of Health's Community Child Health Service (CCHS) [10]. The program uses hemoglobin electrophoresis to test cord blood samples. A pilot program funded by the SickKids Caribbean Initiative using HPLC testing of heel prick samples had a disappointing uptake and the initial approach continues. The pilot in Tobago has also been successful; it has been continuous for a decade. It is funded by the Regional Health Authority of Tobago, which has made the diagnosis and treatment of SCD a priority. Screening of the immediate family of babies identified with the trait or the disease is done by electrophoresis in the hospital laboratory, thus a greater percentage of the population now know their genotype and there is a greater awareness through education. The initiation of SCD NBS at a major obstetric hospital in Trinidad in 2018 is further evidence of the acceptance of this program.

Pilot screening projects in Grenada [13], St Vincent and the Grenadines [17], and Haiti [18], funded by CAREST, the Medical University of South Carolina (Charleston, SC, USA), and University Hospitals Medical Center (Cleveland, OH, USA), respectively, were not sustained once project funding ended. Local policy makers were not able to identify funding and human resources for continued screening. A pilot posited in Barbados was not undertaken [19]. Instead, screening of pregnant women and testing postnatally of at risk children was the approach chosen.

Currently, champions in Antigua and Guyana are pressing to start pilots and perhaps sustainable programs. These outcomes again indicate the importance of advocacy in convincing policy makers of the feasibility and benefit of SCD NBS. In both Jamaica and Saint Lucia, advocacy groups have been critical to convincing public health officials to initiate and maintain screening. CAREST has a role in supporting their advocacy efforts to secure governmental support and sustainable funding, even as screening begins. In this framework, CAREST has recently obtained funding from the European Regional Development Fund. This funding dedicated to the development of cooperation between the French Departments of the Americas and the other countries/territories of the Caribbean Basin will allow the screening of Grenada to be re-launched, initiate a pilot study for Antigua, and evaluate strategies to ensure the sustainability of this NBS.

The Saint-Lucia and Tobago experience clearly demonstrate that the model of using a few regional laboratories to increase efficiencies of scale, decreasing per cost tests, can be used. Actually, given the high cost of equipment and requisite disposables, and the relatively small populations in the Region, the use of two regional laboratories (Jamaica and Guadeloupe) proved to be a cost-effective approach, once reasonably costed transportation of samples and secure data flows are available. However, it is worthwhile to notice that a significant proportion of the Caribbean populations do not have access to screening program, such as Haiti, which accounts for more than 90% the Francophone inhabitants of the Caribbean, and the Dominican Republic, with approximately 40% of Spanish-speakers. Up to now, only a little more than 50% of the English and Spanish speaking infants are screened.

The cost of national SCD NBS programmes may decrease significantly if efficient, accurate, and inexpensive point-of-care (POC) devices become available; a number of such POC testing devices have recently been developed [20]. These low-cost devices, which must have high specificity to detect HbS and HbC in the presence of HbF and the capacity to distinguish the trait (HbAS) from samples with SCD, must also be easy to use. Two of them, relying on lateral flow immunoassays, the SickleSCAN [21] and the HemoTypeSC tests [22], could be viable screening tools for the early diagnosis of SCD conducted by health workers with little expertise. Preliminary data using the HemoTypeSC test on a small series of children and adults in Martinique, in comparison with a larger series in Ghana and the USA, showed the good specificity and sensitivity of the test [23]. We plan to conduct larger studies to evaluate the performance and implementation feasibility of these POC testing devices as screening tools in Caribbean territories where the reference "gold-standard" tests, IEF, and HPLC are not available. This approach may also reduce the number of samples to be screened by the reference laboratories and the delay between the blood sampling and the transmission of the result and ultimately reduce the age of inclusion of the newly identified children. Mothers would get immediate feedback if their children's tests are normal, and be advised of the need to do confirmatory tests in cases consistent with traits or SCD. This promising strategy is expected to promote the extension of screening programs, and lead to the clarification of the prevalence and to a better management of SCD in the Caribbean. Audits of important outcomes, such as time to enrollment in clinic, initiation of splenic palpation, and Pneumococcal prophylaxis, as well as continued ongoing ascertainment of survival in countries and territories with SCD NBS, will help to determine what implementation models are most successful and guide the subsequent initiation of programs in other settings.

Differences of SCD prevalence in the Caribbean islands could be observed, with the highest being detected in Jamaica and Grenada and the lowest in Cuba. Various factors may explain these variations, such as the selective introduction of crop production requiring a greater or lesser need for slaves, the settlement policy of the colonial powers with France and the United Kingdom importing few of their own population compared to Spain, for example, as well as the significance of migrations after the end of slavery (ranging from 1804 in Haiti to 1888 in Brazil). In addition, various β^S/β^C ratios have been detected in the studied populations. Since the distribution of the β^C allele is more restricted than that of the β^S allele in Africa, this data could be related to differences in the African origins of the deported slaves in these territories. These differences in the β^S/β^C ratio could also result from sampling effects; a relatively small number of newborns were screened in some populations. Few epidemiological data from continental countries of the Western coast of the Caribbean Sea coast have been produced so far. An NBS pilot study was conducted in Costa Rica with a total of 70,943 samples and led to the identification of five SS and one SC children [24]. In addition, several clinical reports or genetic studies indicating the presence of SCD in Panama [25], Colombia [26], and Venezuela [27] have been published, but none of these countries have implemented an NBS program on SCD and no accurate data of the prevalence of the disease are available so far, to the best of our knowledge.

In summary, SCD is a perfect example of a disease which fulfils all requirements for doing NBS. Parents are usually asymptomatic and may not know of their risk. Tests done on an asymptomatic baby can allow them to access interventions that decrease morbidity and preventable mortality. CAREST will continue to advocate and work towards universal SCD NBS across the Caribbean Region, regardless of language, per capita income, or political system.

Author Contributions: Conceptualization: M.R., M.-D.H.-D., B.M.-T., and J.K.-M.; Methodology: M.R., L.K., K.L., N.E., G.E., M.E.-J., B.M.-T., M.-D.H.-D., and J.K.-M.; Resources: L.K., K.L., N.E., G.E., M.E.-J., B.M.-T., M.A., and N.K.; Writing-Original Draft Preparation: M.R., J.K.-M., B.M.-T., and M.-D.H.-D.; Writing-Review & Editing: M.R., M.-D.H.-D., L.K., K.L., J.K.-M., B.M.-T., M.A., N.E., G.E., and N.K.; Project administration: M.-D.H.-D., and J.K.-M.

Funding: Funding was provided by the regional councils of Guadeloupe and Martinique, and the general council of Guadeloupe. Funding in Jamaica was provided by the Ministry of Health, the National Health Fund. Equipment was provided by the Brazilian Government and Sagicor. The SickKids Caribbean Initiative funded the SCD NBS coordinator in Jamaica and the St Lucia pilot.

Acknowledgments: The authors wish to acknowledge the contribution of the team of the diagnostic laboratory of hemoglobinopathies of the University Hospital of Guadeloupe for its implication in the NBS of Tobago and Grenada.

Conflicts of Interest: The authors declare no conflict of interest.

References

1. Curtin, P.D. Distribution in space: The colonies of the North Europeans. In *The Atlantic Slave Trade: A Census*; University of Wisconsin Press: Madison, WI, USA, 1969; pp. 51–94.
2. Herrick, J.B. Peculiar elongated and sickle-shaped red blood cell corpuscules in a case of severe anemia. *Arch. Intern. Med.* **1910**, *6*, 517–521. [CrossRef]
3. Serjeant, G.; Serjeant, B.E.; Forbes, M.; Hayes, R.J.; Higgs, D.R.; Lehmann, H. Haemoglobin gene frequencies in the Jamaican population: A study in 100,000 newborns. *Br. J. Haematol.* **1986**, *64*, 253–262. [CrossRef] [PubMed]
4. Kato, G.J.; Piel, F.B.; Reid, C.D.; Gaston, M.H.; Ohene-Frempong, K.; Krishnamurti, L.; Smith, W.R.; Panepinto, J.A.; Weatherall, D.J.; Costa, F.F.; et al. Sickle cell disease. *Nat. Rev. Dis. Primers* **2018**, *4*, 18010. [CrossRef] [PubMed]
5. King, L.; Fraser, R.; Forbes, M.; Grindley, M.; Ali, S.; Reid, M. Newborn sickle cell disease screening: The Jamaican experience (1995–2006). *J. Med. Screen.* **2007**, *14*, 117–122. [CrossRef] [PubMed]
6. Saint-Martin, C.; Romana, M.; Bibrac, A.; Brudey, K.; Tarer, V.; Divialle-Doumdo, L.; Petras, M.; Keclard-Christophe, L.; Lamothe, S.; Broquere, C.; et al. Universal newborn screening for haemoglobinopathies in Guadeloupe (French West Indies): A 27-year experience. *J. Med. Screen.* **2013**, *20*, 177–182. [CrossRef]
7. Heredero-Baute, L. Community-based program for the diagnosis and prevention of genetic disorders in Cuba. Twenty years of experience. *Community Genet.* **2004**, *7*, 130–136. [CrossRef]
8. Svarch, E.; Machín García, S.; Marcheco Teruel, B.; Triana, R.M.; González Otero, A.; Menéndez Veitía, A. Program for comprehensive sickle cell disease care in Cuba. *Revista Cubana de Hematología, Inmunología y Hemoterapia* **2017**, *33*, 1–2.
9. Knight-Madden, J.; Romana, M.; Villaescusa, R.; Reid, M.; Etienne-Julan, M.; Boutin, L.; Elana, G.; Elenga, N.; Wheeler, G.; Lee, K.; et al. CAREST—Multilingual Regional Integration for Health Promotion and Research on Sickle Cell Disease and Thalassemia. *Am. J. Public Health* **2016**, *106*, 851–853. [CrossRef]
10. Alexander, S.; Belmar-George, S.; Eugene, A.; Elias, V. Knowledge of an attitudes toward heel prick screening for sickle cell disease in Saint Lucia. *Rev. Panam. Salud Publica* **2017**, *41*, e70.
11. Kéclard, L.; Romana, M.; Lavocat, E.; Saint-Martin, C.; Berchel, C.; Mérault, G. Sickle cell disorder, beta-globin gene cluster haplotypes and alpha-thalassemia in neonates and adults from Guadeloupe. *Am. J. Hematol.* **1997**, *55*, 24–27. [CrossRef]
12. Romana, M.; Kéclard, L.; Froger, A.; Lavocat, E.; Saint-Martin, C.; Berchel, C.; Mérault, G. Diverse genetic mechanisms operate to generate atypical betaS haplotypes in the population of Guadeloupe. *Hemoglobin* **2000**, *24*, 77–87. [CrossRef] [PubMed]
13. Antoine, M.; Lee, K.; Donald, T.; Belfon, Y.; Drigo, A.; Polson, S.; Martin, F.; Mitchell, G.; Etienne-Julan, M.; Hardy-Dessources, M.D. Prevalence of sickle cell disease among Grenadian newborns. *J. Med. Screen.* **2018**, *25*, 49–50. [CrossRef] [PubMed]
14. Available online: https://www.has-sante.fr/portail/upload/.../ald_10_pnds_drepano_enfant_web.pdf (accessed on 2 April 2010).

15. Aldred, K.; Asnani, M.; Beckford, M.; Bhatt-Poulose, K.; Bortolusso Ali, S.; Chin, N.; Daley, C.; Grindley, M.; Hammond-Gabbadon, C.; Harris, J.; et al. *Sickle Cell Disease: The Clinical Care Guidelines of the Sickle Cell Unit*; Bortolusi-Ali, S., Ed.; Sickle Cell Unit, Tropical Medicine Research Institute, University of the West Indies: Kingston, Jamaica, 2016.
16. Morales, A.; Wierenga, A.; Cuthbert, C.; Sacharow, S.; Jayakar, P.; Velazquez, D.; Loring, J.; Barbouth, D. Expanded newborn screening in Puerto Rico and the US Virgin Islands: Education and barriers assessment. *Genet. Med.* **2009**, *11*, 169–175. [CrossRef] [PubMed]
17. Williams, S.A.; Browne-Ferdinand, B.; Smart, Y.; Morella, K.; Reed, S.G.; Kanter, J. Newborn Screening for Sickle Cell Disease in St. Vincent and the Grenadines: Results of a Pilot Newborn Screening Program. *Glob. Pediatr. Health* **2017**, *4*. [CrossRef]
18. Rotz, S.; Arty, G.; Dall'Amico, R.; De Zen, L.; Zanolli, F.; Bodas, P. Prevalence of sickle cell disease, hemoglobin S, and hemoglobin C among Haitian newborns. *Am. J. Hematol.* **2013**, *88*, 827–828. [CrossRef] [PubMed]
19. Quimby, K.R.; Moe, S.; Sealy, I.; Nicholls, C.; Hambleton, I.R.; Landis, R.C. Clinical findings associated with homozygous sickle cell disease in the Barbadian population–do we need a national SCD registry? *BMC Res. Notes* **2014**, *7*, 102. [CrossRef] [PubMed]
20. McGann, P.T.; Hoppe, C. The pressing need for point-of-care diagnostics for sickle cell disease: A review of current and future technologies. *Blood Cells Mol. Dis.* **2017**, *67*, 104–113. [CrossRef]
21. Nwegbu, M.M.; Isa, H.A.; Nwankwo, B.B.; Okeke, C.C.; Edet-Offong, U.J.; Akinola, N.O.; Adekile, A.D.; Aneke, J.C.; Okocha, E.C.; Ulasi, T.; et al. Preliminary Evaluation of a Point-of-Care Testing Device (SickleSCAN™) in Screening for Sickle Cell Disease. *Hemoglobin* **2017**, *41*, 77–82. [CrossRef]
22. Quinn, C.T.; Paniagua, M.C.; DiNello, R.K.; Panchal, A.; Geisberg, M. A rapid, inexpensive and disposable point-of-care blood test for sickle cell disease using novel, highly specific monoclonal antibodies. *Br. J. Haematol.* **2016**, *175*, 724–732. [CrossRef]
23. Steele, C.; Sinski, A.; Asibey, J.; Hardy-Dessources, M.D.; Elana, G.; Brennan, C.; Odame, I.; Hoppe, C.; Geisberg, M.; Serrao, E.; et al. Point-of-care screening for sickle cell disease in low-resource settings: A multi-center evaluation of HemoTypeSC, a novel rapid test. *Am. J. Hematol.* **2018**. [CrossRef]
24. Abarca, G.; Navarrete, M.; Trejos, R.; de Céspedes, C.; Saborío, M. Abnormal haemoglobins in the newborn human population of Costa Rica. *Rev. Biol. Trop.* **2008**, *56*, 995–1001. [PubMed]
25. Rusanova, I.; Cossio, G.; Moreno, B.; Javier Perea, F.; De Borace, R.G.; Perea, M.; Escames, G.; Acuña-Castroviejo, D. β-globin gene cluster haplotypes in sickle cell patients from Panamá. *Am. J. Hum. Biol.* **2011**, *23*, 377–380. [CrossRef] [PubMed]
26. Fong, C.; Lizarralde-Iragorri, M.A.; Rojas-Gallardo, D.; Barreto, G. Frequency and origin of haplotypes associated with the beta-globin gene cluster in individuals with trait and sickle cell anemia in the Atlantic and Pacific coastal regions of Colombia. *Genet. Mol. Biol.* **2013**, *36*, 494–497. [CrossRef] [PubMed]
27. Arends, A.; Alvarez, M.; Velázquez, D.; Bravo, M.; Salazar, R.; Guevara, J.M.; Castillo, O. Determination of beta-globin gene cluster haplotypes and prevalence of alpha-thalassemia in sickle cell anemia patients in Venezuela. *Am. J. Hematol.* **2000**, *64*, 87–90. [CrossRef]

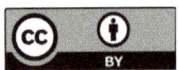

© 2019 by the authors. Licensee MDPI, Basel, Switzerland. This article is an open access article distributed under the terms and conditions of the Creative Commons Attribution (CC BY) license (http://creativecommons.org/licenses/by/4.0/).

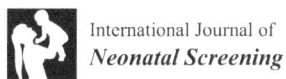
International Journal of
Neonatal Screening

Review

The Neonatal Screening Program in Brazil, Focus on Sickle Cell Disease (SCD)

Ana C. Silva-Pinto [1,2,*], Maria Cândida Alencar de Queiroz [2], Paula Juliana Antoniazzo Zamaro [3], Miranete Arruda [1,4] and Helena Pimentel dos Santos [1,5]

1. Policy of Integral Attention to People with Sickle Cell Disease (PIAPSCD), Technical Advisory Council for Sickle Cell Disease (TAC-SCD), CGSH/DAET/SAS, Ministry of Health, Asa Norte Brasília 70719-040, Brazil; miranetearruda1@gmail.com (M.A.); helena.pimentel@apaesalvador.org.br (H.P.d.S.)
2. Regional Blood Center of Ribeirão Preto, HC-FMRP, University of Sao Paulo (USP), Campus Universitário, Ribeirão Preto 14049-900, Brazil; maria.candida@saude.gov.br
3. National Newborn Screening Program Policy (NNSPP)/CGSH/SAS, Ministry of Health, Asa Norte Brasília 70719-040, Brazil; triagemneonatal@saude.gov.br
4. State Health Secretariat, State of Pernambuco, Recife 50751-530, Brazil
5. Newborn Screening Program, APAE-Salvador, Salvador 41830-141, Brazil
* Correspondence: acristina@hemocentro.fmrp.usp.br; Tel.: +55-162101-9300

Received: 28 September 2018; Accepted: 23 January 2019; Published: 26 January 2019

Abstract: Since 2001, the Brazilian Ministry of Health has been coordinating a National Neonatal Screening Program (NNSP) that now covers all the 26 states and the Federal District of the Brazilian Republic and targets six diseases including sickle cell disease (SCD) and other hemoglobinopathies. In 2005, the program coverage reached 80% of the total live births. Since then, it has oscillated between 80% and 84% globally with disparities from one state to another (>95% in São Paulo State). The Ministry of Health has also published several Guidelines for clinical follow-up and treatment for the diseases comprised by the neonatal screening program. The main challenge was, and still is, to organize the public health network (SUS), from diagnosis and basic care to reference centers in order to provide comprehensive care for patients diagnosed by neonatal screening, especially for SCD patients. Considerable gains have already been achieved, including the implementation of a network within SUS and the addition of scientific and technological progress to treatment protocols. The goals for the care of SCD patients are the intensification of information provided to health care professionals and patients, measures to prevent complications, and care and health promotion, considering these patients in a global and integrated way, to reduce mortality and enhance their quality of life.

Keywords: neonatal screening; sickle cell disease; hemoglobinopathies

1. Background

The Brazilian population is currently estimated at over 208 million people. For the most part, three distinct peoples form the ethnic backgrounds of this population: the Native Americans (Indians), the Portuguese, and the Africans. Population data from the 2010 Demographic Census showed that 50.7% of the Brazilian population is made up of Afro-Americans, 47.7% Caucasians, and 0.7% Indians (0.9% unspecified). Since the population is broadly miscegenated, all national programs must be universalized and not directed at a specific portion of the population. Therefore, the neonatal screening program is national and universal, aiming to reach 100% of live births in the country [1].

2. The Neonatal Screening Program

The history of neonatal screening (NS) in Brazil goes back to 1976, when APAE-São Paulo began neonatal screening for phenylketonuria (PKU). Several pilot NS initiatives were then initiated independently without coordination nor standardization among Brazilian states. In 1992, the screening for PKU and congenital hypothyroidism (CH) was included in the public health system, known as SUS [2]. In 1998, the State of Minas Gerais was the first to introduce a universal State NS Program for sickle cell disease (SCD) in the already existing programs for PK and CH [3].

However, the recognition of NS as a specific public health program only happened in 2001 after the founding of the National Neonatal Screening Program (NNSP) coordinated by the Ministry of Health [4]. The program led to the definition of standards and protocols for the whole country, and placed screening as a global health action aimed at preventing child health problems not only through testing to detect the disease but also the active search of suspected cases, diagnostic confirmation, treatment, and follow-up of patients [5]. The NNSP initially focused on PKU, CH, cystic fibrosis, SCD, and other hemoglobinopathies. In 2014, the program was extended to screening for biotinidase deficiency and congenital adrenal hyperplasia.

The Ministry of Health defined priorities and divided the program into four phases, accrediting the states according to each one's capacity. From 2001 onward, reference services were certified sequentially in one of the four phases of the NNSP. Table 1 shows the years at which each of the phases reached universal implementation in all the states and the Federal District.

Figure 1 illustrates the sequential expansion of the neonatal screening program in the various states of Brazil between 2010 and 2014.

Table 1. The implementation of neonatal screening divided into phases, and its year of universalization.

Phases	Diseases	Year of National Implementation
Phase I	Phenylketonuria and congenital hypothyroidism	2006
Phase II	Sickle cell disease and other hemoglobinopathies	2013
Phase III	Cystic fibrosis	2013
Phase IV	Congenital adrenal hyperplasia and biotinidase deficiency	2014

The coverage rate of the program (percentage of the screened live births) varied over the years (Figure 2). Since 2006, it has remained above 85% at the national level, with few variations. This figure relates to variations in the health care network capacity from state to state and to variations in the population's access to it. In São Paulo State, for example, the percentage of coverage reaches over 95%.

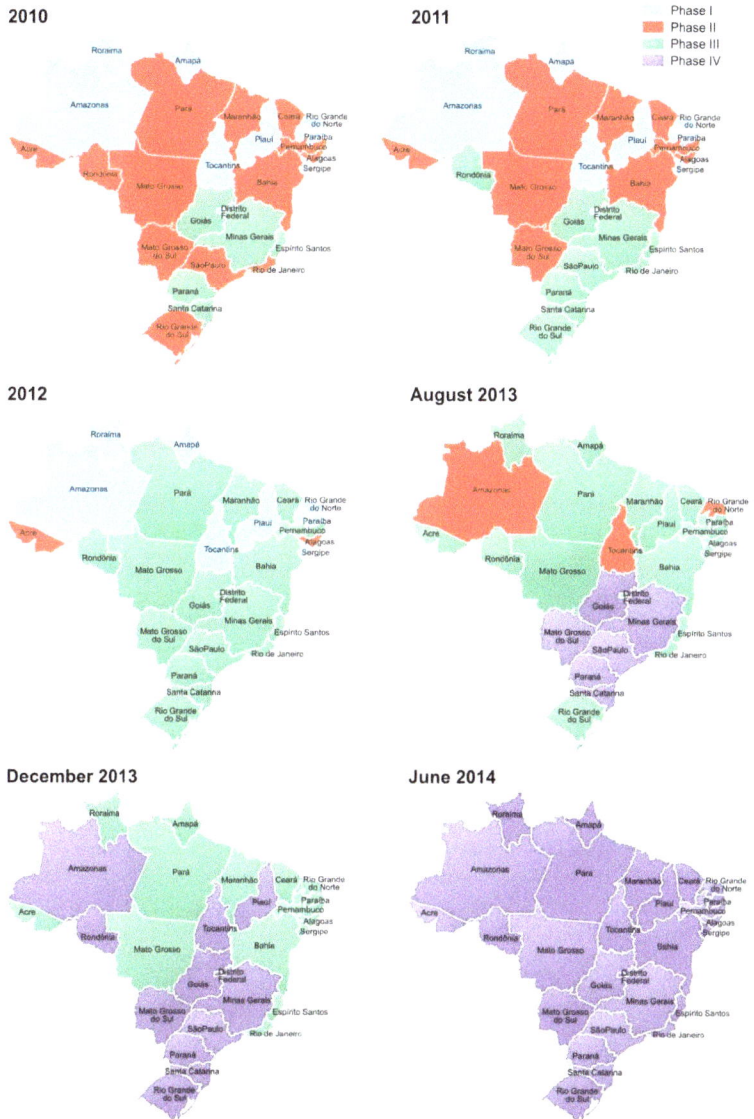

Figure 1. Expansion of the neonatal screening program in Brazil from 2010 to 2014 regarding the four phases of the National Neonatal Screening Program (NNSP).

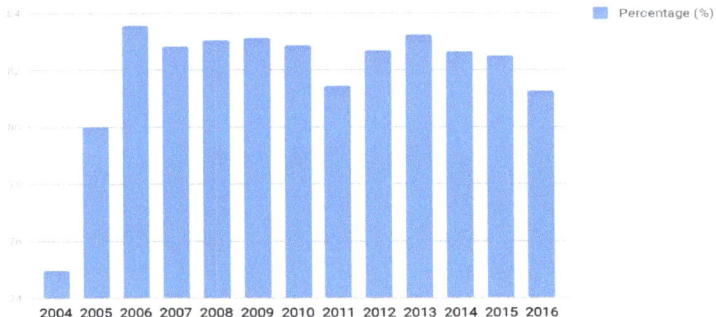

Figure 2. The annual rate of the program coverage from 2004 to 2016.

3. Resolutions and Guidelines from the Brazilian Ministry of Health

In addition to the implementation of neonatal screening and with the goal of standardizing standards of care, the Ministry of Health has published several guidelines for clinical follow-up and treatment for each of the diseases included in the neonatal screening program (see, for example, the Clinical Protocol and Therapeutic Guidelines for Sickle Cell Disease [6]). These include the description of the general concepts for each disease, diagnostic criteria, inclusion and exclusion criteria, treatment and mechanisms of regulation, and control and treatment evaluation. Altogether, they establish a national policy and should be used by the state and municipal Health Secretariats for the regulation of care access, authorization, registration, and reimbursement of the corresponding procedures.

4. The Sickle Cell Disease Network of Care Inside SUS: From Neonatal Screening to Follow-Up in Reference Centers

Health is inscribed in the national Constitution as a right for everyone and a duty of the Brazilian Republic. This was the framework for the creation of the Unified Health System, known as SUS, which contemplates the guidelines for health promotion and provision of services and establishes the community participation and transfer of federal resources to other jurisdictions [7,8]. Despite the great barriers that SUS has faced since its conception, it has managed to establish itself as a system that proposes to be an institutional redistributive model, guaranteeing universal coverage. In this context, the inclusion of sickle cell disease (SCD) and other hemoglobinopathies in the National Neonatal Screening Program (NNSP) instituted by the SUS in 2001 shows recognition of this group of pathologies as a national public health issue [9].

The proportion of live births with SCD varies widely among the states, being more frequent in states with a higher concentration of African descendants. For example, in Bahia for every 650 births, 1 child has SCD, followed by Rio de Janeiro (1:1200) and then Pernambuco, Maranhão, and Minas Gerais, with 1:1400. Table 2 shows the incidence of newborns affected by SCD in 12 states representative of the four most populated regions of Brazil (the fifth region being the North that covers the Amazonian forest).

Table 2. Incidence of sickle cell disease and sickle cell trait in some Brazilian states.

Regions of Brazil	State	Incidence/Live Births	Incidence of the S Mutation
Northeast	Maranhão	1:1400	1:23
Northeast	Pernambuco	1:1400	1:23
Northeast	Bahia	1:650	1:17
Center-west	Goiás	1:1400	1:28
Center-west	Mato Grosso do Sul	1:8300	1:70
Southeast	Minas Gerais	1:1400	1:30
Southeast	Espírito Santo	1:1800	1:28
Southeast	Rio de Janeiro	1:1200	1:21
Southeast	São Paulo	1:4000	1:35
South	Paraná	1:13,000	1:65
South	Santa Catarina	1:13,000	1:65
South	Rio Grande do Sul	1:13,500	1:65

Building up the current network and system of care for the people with SCD in Brazil has been a long process, in some ways reminiscent of the 1970s struggle for civil rights and equality for access to care in the USA that led to the US *National Sickle Cell Anemia Control Act* in 1972 [10,11]. In the 1980s, Brazilian representative entities for the the defense of the rights of family and people with SCD took the first steps to formulate claims, initially at the local level, and then expanded their coordination with the formation in 2001 of the National Federation of Associations of People with Sickle Diseases (FENAFAL). The march Zumbi dos Palmares against Racism, for Citizenship and for Life, held in Brasilia in 1995, was an important milestone in the struggle of black people against the Brazilian State for affirmative action and against racism in terms of health care. From this action, important policies emerged, including the Policy of Integral Attention to People with Sickle Cell Disease (PIAPSCD) [12]. The major goals were to change the natural history of SCD in Brazil, by reducing morbidity and mortality, promoting greater survival, and improving the quality of life for people with SCD. Commitments were made to provide genetic guidance, safeguarding reproductive rights of people with the sickle cell trait, and to disseminate information about SCD to the general population.

In 2006, the Ministry of Health established a Technical Advisory Council for Sickle Cell Disease (TAC-SCD) to help states and municipalities organize their programs of care for people with SCD. TAC is composed of specialists, managers of state and municipal jurisdictions of SUS, and representatives of educational, research, and assistance institutions involved in the care of people with SCD who are invited to act voluntarily. There is also a representation of the users chosen by FENAFAL. TAC is responsible for producing the guidelines for the management of SCD and its complications, genetic guidelines, family guidelines, guidelines for oral health and on the role of nursing, which are printed and distributed in the reference centers and in the basic SUS network. These materials are available electronically in the SUS Virtual Library (VL). The members of TAC also conduct training courses, workshops, and symposia on SCD in all regions of the country, contributing to the continuing education of health professionals.

Within SUS, the standardized attention to people with SCD encompasses all levels from early diagnosis to bone marrow transplantation. Assistance begins in basic care with the early diagnosis free of charge through the NNSP that links the affected child to the basic health unit, responsible for the first procedures of prevention such as prophylaxis with penicillin initiated in the first month of life, immunobiological approaches, and then referral to the regional Specialized Care Service. In most states, the reference center is the Blood Center, which is normally integrated with the local health network to meet other health needs, such as the use of hydroxyurea, transcranial Doppler, and all procedures of greater complexity. The implementation of the SCD network in all the states is intended to guarantee decentralized care beginning with diagnosis, with the assistance of a multi-professional and multidisciplinary team, providing health education with a focus on self-management and access to specialized and high complexity care in all the 26 states and the Federal District [13].

5. Challenges for the Full Implementation of the SCD Care Network

Despite major advances, the organization of a robust health care network for people with SCD is still a major challenge to SUS. Only a network with the potential for the collective construction of solutions is able to cope with the complexity of demands and to guarantee the promotion of autonomy and citizenship to people with SCD. The disease has not yet reached the level of visibility pursued that is necessary to provide its target population with the right to health they deserve to extend their life horizon with personal and social well-being.

Notably, considerable gains have already been achieved, including the implementation of neonatal screening at the national level together with scientific and technological progress with respect to treatment. Preliminary data on the effect of hydroxyurea treatment and mortality rates have been published [14–16]. However, more precise epidemiological data covering the entire country are still needed. A national registry for SCD patients is being set up to collect more reliable information to evaluate the system: percentage of new cases that actually enter follow-up at reference centers, immunization rate, percentage of patients that started pneumococcal prophylaxis, rate of children screened with transcranial Doppler, use of hydroxyurea, and death rates at the country level. What is sought to bring attention to people with SCD is the intensification of information provided, measures to prevent injuries, and care and health promotion, considering these patients in a global and integrated way, to reduce mortality and enhance their quality of life.

Author Contributions: All authors contributed equally to the manuscript: A.C.S.-P. was responsible for the design, writing, and review of the manuscript; M.C.A.d.Q. was responsible for the SCD network writing and review; P.J.A.Z. was responsible for the newborn screening data and figures; M.A. was responsible for SCD epidemiological data and the review of the final version; and H.P.d.S. was responsible for the newborn screening background and review of the manuscript.

Funding: This research received no external funding.

Conflicts of Interest: The authors declare no conflict of interest.

References

1. Brasil, IBGE. Demographic Census 2010. Available online: https://www.ibge.gov.br/ (accessed on 17 September 2018).
2. Brasil, Ministério da Saúde. Portaria GM/MS n°22 de 15/01/1992—triagem para fenilcetonúria e hipotireoidismo Congênito. *Diário Oficial da União*, 15 January 1992.
3. Paixão, M.C.; Cunha Ferraz, M.H.; Januário, J.N.; Viana, M.B.; Lima, J.M. Reliability of isoelectrofocusing for the detection of Hb S, Hb C, and HB D in a pioneering population-based program of newborn screening in Brazil. *Hemoglobin* **2001**, *25*, 297–303. [CrossRef] [PubMed]
4. Brasil, Ministério da saúde. Portaria GM/MS n° 822 de 06 de junho de 2001—Programa de triagem neonatal no Brasil. *Diário Oficial da União*, 6 June 2001.
5. Carvalho, T.M.; Santos, H.P.; Santos, I.C.G.P.; Vargas, P.R.; Pedrosa, J. Newborn screening: A national public health programme in Brazil. *J. Inherit. Metab. Dis.* **2007**, *30*, 615. [CrossRef] [PubMed]
6. Brasil, Ministério da saúde. Portaria SAS/MS N° 55 de 29 de janeiro de 2010—Protocolo Clínico e Diretrizes Terapêuticas para Doença Falciforme". *Diário Oficial da União*, 29 January 2010.
7. Brasil, Ministério da saúde. Lei n° 8.080, de 19 de setembro de 1990, criação do SUS—Sistema Único de Saúde. *Diário Oficial da União*, 19 September 1990.
8. Seta, M.H.; Oliveira, C.V.D.S.; Pepe, V.L.E. Health protection in Brazil: the National Sanitary Surveillance System. *Cien Saude Colet* **2017**, *22*, 3225–3234. [CrossRef] [PubMed]
9. Ramalho, A.S.; Magna, L.A.; Paiva-Silva, R.B. A portaria n° 822/01 do Ministério da Saúde e as peculiaridades das hemoglobinopatias em saúde pública no Brasil. *Cad. Saúde Pública* **2003**, *19*, 1195–1199. [CrossRef] [PubMed]

10. Vichinsky, E. Sickle cell disease and thalassemia: disorders of globin production. (2008) pages 3-5, in Special anniversary brochure, American Society of Hematology: 50 Years in Hematology: Research That Revolutionized Patient Care. Available online: http://www.hematology.org/About/History/50-Years/1533.aspx (accessed on 13 January 2019).
11. Bassett, M.T. Beyond Berets: The Black Panthers as Health Activists. *Am. J. Public Health* **2016**, *106*, 1741–1743. [CrossRef] [PubMed]
12. Brasil, Ministério da saúde. Portaria de n° 1391 de 16 de agosto de 2005—Diretrizes para a Política Nacional de Atenção Integral às Pessoas com Doença Falciforme e outras Hemoglobinopatias. *Diário Oficial da União*, 16 August 2005.
13. Cançado, R.D.; Jesus, J.A. A doença falciforme no Brasil. *Rev. Bras. Hematol. Hemoter.* **2007**, *29*, 204–206. [CrossRef]
14. Lobo, C.L.; Pinto, J.F.; Nascimento, E.M.; Moura, P.G.; Cardoso, G.P.; Hankins, J.S. The effect of hydroxcarbamide therapy on survival of children with sickle cell disease. *Br. J. Haematol.* **2013**, *161*, 852–860. [CrossRef] [PubMed]
15. Fernandes, A.P.; Januário, J.N.; Cangussu, C.B.; Macedo, D.L.; Viana, M.B. Mortality of children with sickle cell disease: A population study. *J. Pediatr. (Rio J).* **2010**, *86*, 279–284. [CrossRef]
16. Lobo, C.L.C.; Nascimento, E.M.D.; Jesus, L.J.C.; Freitas, T.G.; Lugon, J.R.; Ballas, S.K. Mortality in children, adolescents and adults with sickle cell anemia in Rio de Janeiro, Brazil. *Rev. Bras. Hematol. Hemoter.* **2018**, *40*, 37–42. [CrossRef] [PubMed]

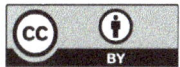

© 2019 by the authors. Licensee MDPI, Basel, Switzerland. This article is an open access article distributed under the terms and conditions of the Creative Commons Attribution (CC BY) license (http://creativecommons.org/licenses/by/4.0/).

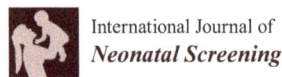

Review

Newborn Screening for Sickle Cell Disease: Indian Experience

Roshan B. Colah, Pallavi Mehta and Malay B. Mukherjee *

ICMR-National Institute of Immunohaematology, KEM Hospital Campus, Mumbai 400012, India; colahrb@gmail.com (R.B.C.); sarthi710@gmail.com (P.M.)
* Correspondence: malaybmukherjee@gmail.com

Received: 12 September 2018; Accepted: 7 November 2018; Published: 13 November 2018

Abstract: Sickle cell disease (SCD) is a major public health problem in India with the highest prevalence amongst the tribal and some non-tribal ethnic groups. The clinical manifestations are extremely variable ranging from a severe to mild or asymptomatic condition. Early diagnosis and providing care is critical in SCD because of the possibility of lethal complications in early infancy in pre-symptomatic children. Since 2010, neonatal screening programs for SCD have been initiated in a few states of India. A total of 18,003 babies have been screened by automated HPLC using either cord blood samples or heel prick dried blood spots and 2944 and 300 babies were diagnosed as sickle cell carriers and SCD respectively. A follow up of the SCD babies showed considerable variation in the clinical presentation in different population groups, the disease being more severe among non-tribal babies. Around 30% of babies developed serious complications within the first 2 to 2.6 years of life. These pilot studies have demonstrated the feasibility of undertaking newborn screening programs for SCD even in rural areas. A longer follow up of these babies is required and it is important to establish a national newborn screening program for SCD in all of the states where the frequency of the sickle cell gene is very high followed by the development of comprehensive care centers along with counselling and treatment facilities. This comprehensive data will ultimately help us to understand the natural history of SCD in India and also help the Government to formulate strategies for the management and prevention of sickle cell disease in India.

Keywords: newborn screening; sickle cell disease; India; tribal; non-tribal; Guthrie spots; cord blood; automated HPLC

1. Introduction

Hemoglobinopathies are the most common monogenic disorders in India posing a significant health burden. Sickle cell disease (SCD) was the first molecular disease to be described where a single point mutation (A→T) resulted in the substitution of the 6th aminoacid in the β globin chain from glutamic acid to valine leading to an altered electrophoretic mobility of the hemoglobin molecule. SCD includes a variety of conditions, the primary hemoglobin disorder being sickle cell anemia (SCA) due to homozygosity for hemoglobin S (HbS) as well as the compound heterozygous conditions, HbS-β thalassemia, HbSD disease, HbSE disease, HbSC disease and HbS-O Arab disease [1].

2. Geographic Distribution of HbS in India

HbS is widespread in African, Mediterranean, Middle Eastern, Indian, Caribbean and South and Central American populations [1]. In India, SCA is prevalent among tribal populations who are considered to be the original inhabitants in south Gujarat, Maharashtra, Madhya Pradesh, Chhattisgarh, and western Odisha with a smaller focus in the southern region in Andhra Pradesh, Karnataka, northern Tamil Nadu and Kerala. They often reside in remote regions away from the mainstream populations. Sickle cell anemia is also prevalent in some of the scheduled castes and other backward classes (non-tribal populations) mainly in central India, in particular, among the Mahar, Kunbi and Teli castes but is rare in other castes where it may be seen due to admixture. These are economically and socially disadvantaged populations living largely in rural areas. Carrier frequencies ranging from 1 to 35% have been described in these groups and their distribution in different states of the country has been mapped earlier [2–4]. Many of these populations also harbor the β thalassemia gene but screening for β thalassemia had not been extensively carried out among them earlier. A recent report from Akola district in central India showed that 36 out of 91 pediatric SCD patients (39.6%) had sickle-β thalassemia [5].

3. Sickle Haplotypes in India

In the eastern province of Saudi Arabia and in India, the sickle gene is linked to the Arab Indian or Asian haplotype, which is associated with higher fetal hemoglobin (HbF) levels and a milder clinical presentation than the Benin haplotype seen in west and north Africa and the Bantu haplotype seen in east and central Africa [6]. There are limited studies on haplotype analysis from different regions in India, however, all of them have shown that around 90% of sickle genes have the Asian haplotype while few other atypical haplotypes including the BantuA2 and the Senegal haplotype have been associated with around 10% of sickle genes [7]. Yet, recent studies have indicated more severe clinical manifestations even among the Asian haplotype.

4. Clinical Manifestations of Sickle Cell Disease in India

Initial studies on sickle cell disease patients from western Odisha demonstrated a mild clinical course with higher hemoglobin levels, lower reticulocyte counts, persistence of splenomegaly, infrequent leg ulcers and priapism compared to patients with the disease of African origin [8]. Subsequently, in western and central India it was found that the disease was milder among tribal populations in Valsad in south Gujarat compared to non-tribal populations in Nagpur in Maharashtra. Apart from higher HbF levels, a significant ameliorating factor was the presence of associated α thalassemia, which was very common in tribal populations in Gujarat [9]. Since then, reports of more severe features, particularly from central India have raised the question of geographic variations in the manifestations of SCD within India. In a retrospective study, where 316 children with sickle cell anemia were followed up for a period of 5.8 ± 5.7 years in Nagpur, there were 1725 hospitalizations among 282 patients and 96 children had severe disease with severe vaso occlusive crises, severe anemia, splenic sequestration, stroke and hypersplenism being reported and 10 babies died during this period [10]. Another retrospective analysis of 110 adult patients with sickle cell disease who attended out-patient clinics or were admitted to the hospital showed that 75.4% of them had a severe disease in spite of all the sickle genes being linked to the Asian haplotype and the presence of associated α thalassemia [11]. Thus, sickle cell disease has an extremely variable clinical presentation in Indian patients.

5. Providing Comprehensive Care in Rural Regions

As a large majority of sickle cell disease cases are born in rural India, it is necessary to provide adequate care for these patients, which can be challenging in remote areas. However, few studies from different regions have demonstrated that this is possible with the involvement of Government and Non-Government Organizations as well as representatives from the local population. It was shown in a study from the Bardoli district in Gujarat that giving basic health care training to a local villager to regularly visit households and monitor sickle cell disease cases and identify those with significant complications and refer them to the coordinating hospital would have a significant impact on tribal communities with a high prevalence of SCD [12]. In another study undertaken in a remote tribal village in Gudalur in south India, it was shown that 71% of 111 patients with sickle cell disease were able to have at least one annual comprehensive care visit. Premature deaths were seen in 19 patients at a median age of 23 years due to acute chest syndrome, sepsis, severe anemia, stroke or sudden unexplained deaths [13]. A comprehensive care model at Sewa Rural in Gujarat was successfully implemented, which included screening, both out-patient and in-patient care of SCD patients as well as health education. A one year follow up of 164 SCD patients in this rural region was possible and pain crises were seen in 72 patients (43.9%); 59 patients (35.9%) required hospitalization, 43 patients (26.2%) required blood transfusions and three patients (1.6%) died during this short follow up [14].

6. Benefits of Newborn Screening and Comprehensive Care

Newborn screening (NBS) enables the identification of babies with sickle cell disease at birth or soon after, within the first few days of their life before they present with any symptoms or complications. These babies can then be regularly followed up with the provision of comprehensive care and timely management to reduce morbidity and mortality. It has been demonstrated in several countries that early diagnosis and providing care is critical in SCD because of the possibility of lethal complications in the first few years of life in pre-symptomatic children. Young children with SCD have an increased susceptibility to bacteremia due to *Streptococcus pneumonia*, which can be fatal in many cases. Acute splenic sequestration crisis is another cause for mortality in infancy. Many studies done globally have shown that early prophylactic penicillin can significantly reduce the morbidity and mortality due to pneumococcal sepsis and they have also shown the importance of pneumococcal vaccines for the prevention of pneumococcal sepsis, thus justifying the need for implementing newborn screening programs for SCD [15,16].

7. Newborn Screening Initiatives in India

It has been estimated that three countries, Nigeria, D R Congo and India are most affected by SCD and widespread newborn screening and follow up care could save the lives of almost 10 million children by 2050. It is also estimated that 15% of the world's neonates with sickle cell anemia are born in India [17]. Thus, newborn screening has a great relevance in this country. There is no National neonatal screening program for SCD as yet and affected children are generally identified when they become symptomatic. However, few newborn screening programs have been initiated in some regions in the last 5 to 6 years. Figure 1 shows the location of the different centers involved in newborn screening programs in India. Table 1 summarizes the programs undertaken in a few states in this vast country.

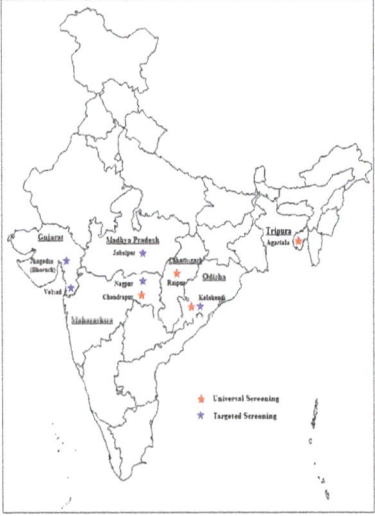

Figure 1. Location of the different centers in India where newborn screening was undertaken.

Table 1. Summary of newborn screening programs initiated in India.

State	District	Target Population	Sample	Technology for Screening	No. Screened	No(%)AS	No(%)SCD	Follow Up	Reference
South Gujarat Phase 1	Valsad	All Tribal babies	Heel prick-Dried blood spot	HPLC-Variant NBS machine	5467	687 (12.5%)	46 (0.8%)	5–6 years	Italia et al., 2015 [18]
South Gujarat Phase 2	Valsad, Bharuch	All Tribal babies	Heel prick-Dried blood spot	HPLC-Variant NBS machine	2944	649 (22.0%)	76 (2.6%)	2 years	Unpublished
Maharashtra	Nagpur	Largely non-tribal, babies of AS mothers	Cord blood, heel prick	HPLC-Variant Hb Testing System	2134	978 (45.8%)	113 (5.3%)	4-5 years	Upadhye et al., 2016 [19]
Madhya Pradesh	Jabalpur	Tribal, babies of AS mothers	Cord blood, heel prick	HPLC-Variant Hb Testing System	461	36 (7.8%)	6 (1.3%)	1 year	Unpublished
Chhattisgarh	Raipur	Tribal and non-tribal babies	Heel prick-Dried blood spot	HPLC-Variant NBS machine	1158	61 (5.3%)	6 (0.5%)	No follow up reported	Panigrahi et al., 2012 [20]
Odisha	Kalahandi	Tribal and non-triba babies	Heel prick-Dried blood spot	HPLC-Variant Hb Testing System	1668	293 (17.6%)	34 (2.0%)	No follow up reported	Mohanty et al., 2010 [21]
Odisha	Kalahandi	Tribal babies	Cord blood	HPLC-Variant Hb Testing System	761	112 (14.7%)	13 (1.7%)	No follow up reported	Dixit et al., 2015 [22]
Tripura	Agartala	Tribal & non tribal babies	Cord blood	HPLC-Variant Hb Testing System	2400	15 (0.6%)	0 (0.0%)	Not done	Upadhye et al., 2018 [23]
Maharashtra	Chandrapur	Tribal and non-tribal babies	Cord blood, heel prick	HPLC-Variant Hb Testing System	1010	85 (8.4%)	4 (0.4%)	Not done	Unpublished

Most of the above were pilot studies undertaken in different states, which showed that it was feasible to undertake newborn screening for SCD even in rural regions and register affected babies for follow up and comprehensive care although the outcome of the follow up was not reported in all these studies.

8. Technologies Used for Newborn Screening in India

Globally, isoelectric focusing (IEF) using eluates from dried blood spots was initially used for screening of newborn babies for sickle cell disease but at many centers this had been replaced by high-performance liquid chromatography (HPLC) analysis [24,25]. In all of the Indian reports on newborn screening for SCD, HPLC analysis has been used. This was mainly due to two reasons. Automated HPLC machines were already in use at these centers for other programs, hence, no additional cost for infrastructure was required. Secondly, it was felt that these machines would be easier to operate and maintain even in rural areas. The Variant NBS machine (BioRad laboratories, Hercules, CA, USA) has been used for hemoglobin analysis from dried blood spots or the Variant Hemoglobin Testing System (BioRad laboratories) for cord blood samples using either the sickle cell short or the β thal short programs. The β thal short program had the advantage of picking up other hemoglobin abnormalities including some rare non-deletional α chain variants like Hb Fontainebleau, Hb O Indonesia and Hb Koya Dora [26]. More recently, several point-of-care devices have been developed for screening, which are either paper-based screening protocols or antibody-based rapid diagnostic devices based on lateral flow immunoassay technologies. They are simple to use and relatively inexpensive as they do not require any specific equipment or even electricity, which is often not always available in remote rural regions. These commercial devices are still being validated for newborn screening for SCD [27,28]. Presently, we are also undertaking a multicenter validation of one of these newborn screening kits to evaluate its suitability for use in newborn screening programs in India in the future.

9. Follow up of Birth Cohorts of Sickle Cell Disease in India

A systematic follow up of SCD babies for around 4 to 5 years had been possible in at least two newborn screening programs in the country in Valsad in south Gujarat and Nagpur in Maharashtra [18,19]. The program in Gujarat targeted mainly tribal newborn babies from four districts. These babies were largely from nine different tribes, the highest numbers being from the Dhodia Patel, Kukna and Halpita tribes. It involved 13 centers (government district hospitals to community health centers) for neonatal sample collection on filter paper. These dried blood spots were sent for processing on the NBS variant machine to the centralized laboratory in Valsad. Of the 5467 babies screened, 687 were identified as sickle cell trait and 46 babies had sickle cell disease (SS-33, S-β-thal-13). After confirmation of the diagnosis, the SCD babies were registered for comprehensive care. Follow up from 1.5 to 5 years was possible only in 32 (69%) of these babies. Pneumococcal vaccination and folic acid supplementation were given to all of the babies. In this cohort, 18 babies (SS-11, S-β thal-7) had no clinical complications till the last follow-up. The majority of the babies who became symptomatic presented after 2 years of age. Seven babies (SS-6, S-β thal-1) had severe complications, which included severe infections, vasoocclusive crises, severe anemia and acute chest syndrome. Few others had mild febrile episodes and mild splenomegaly and hepatomegaly were seen in some babies. One baby died at the age of 4 years during the follow up period. Although haplotyping was not done in all of the SS babies, the Xmn1 polymorphism in 24 SS babies, where this was determined, was Xmn1 (+/+) in all of them. The HbF levels varied from 12.5 to 30.2% among those SS babies who were between 2.4 and 5 years of age. The prevalence of α thalassemia was 92% in this population, the most common α genotype being $-\alpha^{3.7}/-\alpha^{3.7}$ [18]. In the second phase of this program, mobile phones were given to the parents of affected babies to improve compliance for follow ups and this had a significant impact.

In Nagpur in Maharashtra, newborn screening was done at a single government medical college where only babies born to sickle heterozygous mothers were screened making the program more cost-effective. The population here was largely non-tribal, the majority being from the Mahar community. A total of 2134 babies of mothers having a positive solubility test were screened by the collection of cord blood at birth or a heel prick sample subsequently and analyzed by HPLC on the Variant Hemoglobin Testing System. There were 978 babies with sickle cell trait and 113 babies with sickle cell disease (SS-104, S-βthal-7, SD-2). In this cohort too, 73% of the babies could be followed up for 3 to 5 years. Penicillin prophylaxis was given to the babies who could be followed up. Here several babies presented much earlier than the cohort in Gujarat and 45% of the SCD babies required hospitalization between 3 months and 2 years. Infections, severe anemia and painful events were the common presenting features. Eight sickle homozygous babies had sepsis. Six SCD babies died during the follow up period. Haplotyping was done in 75 SS babies and 141 of the 150 SS chromosomes (94%) were linked to the Asian haplotype. Six SS chromosomes were linked to the Bantu A2 haplotype and three to an atypical haplotype. The mean HbF level in the SS cohort was 21.4 ± 5.4%. The prevalence of α thalassemia in this cohort was 28%, the $-\alpha^{3.7}/\alpha\alpha$ genotype being the commonest defect.

Newborn screening for hemoglobinopathies was also undertaken in the malaria endemic northeastern region in Agartala in Tripura where Hb E is widely prevalent but Hb S is also seen among the tea garden workers who are migrant laborers from other states [23]. Only 15 newborn babies with sickle cell trait were identified but 9.3% of babies had HbE trait, 3.3% were Hb E homozygous and one baby had HbE-β thalassemia. Screening for G6PD deficiency was also done and few babies with Hb abnormalities were also G6PD deficient.

The clinical presentation among sickle cell disease babies was quite variable in the two cohorts which could be followed up for at least 4 to 5 years. As mentioned in a recent editorial, the question remains whether the intervention programs developed for African disease could be applied to Indian patients with the Asian haplotype [29]. Newborn cohort studies in different regions in India will be able to answer these questions once they have been systematically undertaken and the affected babies followed up for a longer duration.

10. Lessons Learnt from Pilot Studies on Newborn Screening for Sickle Cell Disease in India

The feasibility of establishing newborn screening programs in tribal areas in rural regions has been shown. Follow up of birth cohorts in the studies where this was done showed that the clinical presentation was very variable in different regions. Further efforts and motivation are needed to ensure that the maximum number of babies can be enrolled and continue to receive comprehensive care and the follow up of babies can be done for a longer duration. Newborn screening programs must be extended to other states where the sickle gene is prevalent. Guidelines for a National Hemoglobinopathy Program have been recently laid down by the Ministry of Health and Family Welfare which also includes newborn screening for SCD and these will be followed for understanding the natural history of sickle cell disease in India [30].

Author Contributions: Conceptualization, R.B.C. and M.B.M.; Data Compilation, R.B.C., P.M. and M.B.M.; Writing—Review and Editing, R.B.C. and M.B.M.

Funding: This review received no external funding.

Acknowledgments: We thank all the investigators associated with these studies.

Conflicts of Interest: The author declares no conflicts of interest.

References

1. Serjeant, G.R.; Serjeant, B.E. (Eds.) *Sickle Cell Disease*; Oxford Medical Publications: New York, NY, USA, 2001.
2. Urade, B.P. Incidence of sickle cell anemia and thalassemia in Central India. *Open J. Blood Dis.* **2012**, *2*, 71–80. [CrossRef]
3. Colah, R.; Mukherjee, M.; Ghosh, K. Sickle cell disease in India. *Curr. Opin. Hematol.* **2014**, *21*, 215–223. [CrossRef] [PubMed]

4. Colah, R.B.; Mukherjee, M.B.; Martin, S.; Ghosh, K. Sickle cell disease in tribal populations in India. *Indian J. Med. Res.* **2015**, *141*, 509–515. [PubMed]
5. Jain, D.; Warthe, V.; Dayama, P.; Sarate, D.; Colah, R.; Mehta, P.; Serjeant, G. Sickle Cell Disease in Central India: A Potentially Severe Syndrome. *Indian J. Pediatr.* **2016**, *83*, 1071–1076. [CrossRef] [PubMed]
6. Pagnier, J.; Mears, J.G.; Dunda-Belkhodja, O.; Schaefer-Rego, K.E.; Beldjord, C.; Nagel, R.L.; Labie, D. Evidence for the multicentric origin of the sickle cell hemoglobin gene in Africa. *Proc. Natl. Acad. Sci. USA* **1984**, *81*, 1771–1773. [CrossRef] [PubMed]
7. Mukherjee, M.B.; Surve, R.R.; Gangakhedkar, R.R.; Ghosh, K.; Colah, R.B.; Mohanty, D. β-globin gene cluster haplotypes linked to the βS gene in western India. *Hemoglobin* **2004**, *28*, 157–161. [CrossRef] [PubMed]
8. Kar, B.C.; Satapathy, R.K.; Kulozik, A.E.; Kulozik, M.; Sirr, S.; Serjeant, B.E.; Serjeant, G.R. Sickle cell disease in Orissa State, India. *Lancet* **1986**, *2*, 1198–1201. [CrossRef]
9. Mukherjee, M.B.; Lu, C.Y.; Ducrocq, R.; Gangakhedkar, R.R.; Colah, R.B.; Kadam, M.D.; Mohanty, D.; Nagel, R.L.; Krishnamoorthy, R. The effect of alpha thalassemia on sickle cell anemia linked to the Arab-Indian haplotype among a tribal and non-tribal population in India. *Am. J. Hematol.* **1997**, *55*, 104–109. [CrossRef]
10. Jain, D.; Italia, K.; Sarathi, V.; Ghosh, K.; Colah, R. Sickle cell anemia from central India: A retrospective analysis. *Indian Pediatr.* **2012**, *49*, 911–913. [CrossRef] [PubMed]
11. Italia, K.; Kangne, H.; Shanmukaiah, C.; Nadkarni, A.H.; Ghosh, K.; Colah, R.B. Variable phenotypes of sickle cell disease in India with the Arab-Indian haplotype. *Br. J. Haematol.* **2015**, *168*, 156–159. [CrossRef] [PubMed]
12. Patel, J.; Patel, B.; Gamit, M.; Serjeant, G.R. Screening for the sickle cell gene in Gujarat, India; a village based model. *J. Community Genet.* **2013**, *4*, 43–47. [CrossRef] [PubMed]
13. Nimgaonkar, V.; Krishnamurti, L.; Prabhakar, H.; Menon, N. Comprehensive integrated care of patients with sickle cell disease in a remote aboriginal tribal population in southern India. *Pediatr. Blood Cancer* **2014**, *61*, 702–705. [CrossRef] [PubMed]
14. Desai, G.; Dave, K.P.; Bannerjee, S.; Barbaria, P.; Gupta, R. Initial outcomes of a comprehensive care model for sickle cell disease among a tribal population in rural western India. *Int. J. Community Med. Public Health* **2016**, *3*, 1282–1287. [CrossRef]
15. Gaston, M.H.; Verter, J.I.; Woods, G.; Pegelow, C.; Kelleher, J.; Presbury, G.; Zarkowsky, H.; Vichinsky, E.; Iyer, R.; Lobel, J.S.; et al. Prophylaxis with oral penicillin in children with sickle cell anemia: A randomized trial. *N. Engl. J. Med.* **1986**, *314*, 1593–1599. [CrossRef] [PubMed]
16. Adamkiewicz, T.V.; Sarnaik, S.; Buchanan, G.R.; Iyer, R.V.; Miller, S.T.; Pegelow, C.H.; Rogers, Z.R.; Vichinsky, E.; Elliott, J.; Facklam, R.R.; et al. Invasive pneumococcal infections in children with sickle cell disease in the era of penicillin prophylaxis, antibiotic resistance, and 23-valent pneumococcal polysaccharide vaccination. *J. Pediatr.* **2003**, *143*, 438–444. [CrossRef]
17. Piel, F.B.; Hay, S.I.; Gupta, S.; Weatherall, D.J.; Williams, T.N. Global burden of sickle cell anaemia in children under five, 2010–2050: Modelling based on demographics, excess mortality, and interventions. *PLoS Med.* **2013**, *10*, e1001484. [CrossRef] [PubMed]
18. Italia, Y.; Krishnamurti, L.; Mehta, V.; Raicha, B.; Italia, K.; Mehta, P.; Ghosh, K.; Colah, R. Feasibility of a Newborn Screening and Follow-up Programme for Sickle Cell Disease among South Gujarat (India) Tribal Populations. *J. Med. Screen.* **2015**, *22*, 1–7. [CrossRef] [PubMed]
19. Upadhye, D.S.; Jain, D.L.; Trivedi, Y.L.; Nadkarni, A.H.; Ghosh, K.; Colah, R.B. Neonatal screening and the clinical outcome in children with sickle cell disease in central India. *PLoS ONE* **2016**, *11*, e0147081. [CrossRef] [PubMed]
20. Panigrahi, S.; Patra, P.K.; Khodiar, P.K. Neonatal screening of sickle cell anemia: A preliminary report. *Indian J. Pediatr.* **2012**, *79*, 747–750. [CrossRef] [PubMed]
21. Mohanty, D.; Das, K.; Mishra, K. Newborn screening for sickle cell disease and congenital hypothyroidism in western Orissa. In Proceedings of the 4th International Congress on Sickle Cell Disease, Raipur, India, 22–27 November 2010; pp. 29–30.
22. Dixit, S.; Sahu, P.; Kar, S.K.; Negi, S. Identification of the hot spot areas for sickle cell disease using cord blood screening at a district hospital: An Indian perspective. *J. Community Genet.* **2015**, *6*, 383–387. [CrossRef] [PubMed]

23. Upadhye, D.; Das, R.; Ray, J.; Acharjee, S.; Ghosh, K.; Colah, R.; Mukherjee, M. Newborn screening for hemoglobinopathies and red cell enzymopathies in Tripura state: A malaria endemic state in Northeast India. *Hemoglobin* **2018**, *42*, 43–46. [CrossRef] [PubMed]
24. Consensus Development Summaries. *Newborn Screening for Sickle Cell Disease and Other Hemoglobinophathies*; Connecticut Medicine; National Institutes of Health: Bethesda, MD, USA, 1987; Volume 51, pp. 459–463.
25. Michlitsch, J.; Azimi, M.; Hoppe, C.; Walters, M.C.; Lubin, B.; Lorey, F.; Vichinsky, E. Newborn screening for hemoglobinopathies in California. *Pediatr. Blood Cancer* **2009**, *52*, 486–490. [CrossRef] [PubMed]
26. Upadhye, D.S.; Jain, D.; Nair, S.B.; Nadkarni, A.H.; Ghosh, K.; Colah, R.B. First case of Hb Fontainebleau with sickle haemoglobin and other non deletional α gene variants identified in neonates during newborn screening for sickle cell disorders. *J. Clin. Pathol.* **2012**, *65*, 654–659. [CrossRef] [PubMed]
27. Piety, N.Z.; George, A.; Serrano, A.; Lanzi, M.R.; Patel, P.R.; Note, M.P.; Kahan, S.; Nirenburg, D.; Camanda, J.F.; Airewale, G.; et al. A paper based test for screening newborns for sickle cell disease. *Sci. Rep.* **2017**, *7*, 45488. [CrossRef] [PubMed]
28. Quinn, C.T.; Paniagua, M.C.; DiNello, R.K.; Panchal, A.; Geisberg, M. A rapid inexpensive and disposable point-of-care blood test for sickle cell disease using novel, highly specific monoclonal antibodies. *Br. J. Haematol.* **2016**, *175*, 724–732. [CrossRef] [PubMed]
29. Serjeant, G.R. Evolving locally appropriate models of care for Indian sickle cell disease. *Indian J. Med. Res.* **2016**, *143*, 405–413. [CrossRef] [PubMed]
30. *National Health Mission Guidelines on Hemoglobinopathies in India*; Ministry of Health and Family Welfare, Government of India: New Delhi, India, 2016.

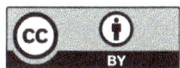

© 2018 by the authors. Licensee MDPI, Basel, Switzerland. This article is an open access article distributed under the terms and conditions of the Creative Commons Attribution (CC BY) license (http://creativecommons.org/licenses/by/4.0/).

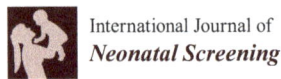

International Journal of
Neonatal Screening

Review

Point-of-Care Testing for G6PD Deficiency: Opportunities for Screening

Athena Anderle [1], Germana Bancone [2,3], Gonzalo J. Domingo [1,*], Emily Gerth-Guyette [1], Sampa Pal [1] and Ari W. Satyagraha [4]

1. PATH, 2201 Westlake Ave, Suite 200, Seattle, WA 98121, USA; aanderle@path.org (A.A.); egerthguyette@path.org (E.G.-G.); spal@path.org (S.P.)
2. Shoklo Malaria Research Unit, Mahidol–Oxford Tropical Medicine Research Unit, Faculty of Tropical Medicine, Mahidol University, 68/30 Bantung Road, PO Box 46 Mae Sot, Tak 63110, Thailand; germana@tropmedres.ac
3. Centre for Tropical Medicine and Global Health, Nuffield Department of Medicine, University of Oxford, Old Road campus, Roosevelt Drive, Oxford OX3 7FZ, UK
4. Eijkman Institute, Jalan Diponegoro 69, Jakarta 10430, Indonesia; ari@eijkman.go.id
* Correspondence: gdomingo@path.org; Tel.: +1-206-302-6741

Received: 1 October 2018; Accepted: 14 November 2018; Published: 19 November 2018

Abstract: Glucose-6-phosphate dehydrogenase (G6PD) deficiency, an X-linked genetic disorder, is associated with increased risk of jaundice and kernicterus at birth. G6PD deficiency can manifest later in life as severe hemolysis, when the individual is exposed to oxidative agents that range from foods such as fava beans, to diseases such as typhoid, to medications such as dapsone, to the curative drugs for *Plasmodium* (*P*.) *vivax* malaria, primaquine and tafenoquine. While routine testing at birth for G6PD deficiency is recommended by the World Health Organization for populations with greater than 5% prevalence of G6PD deficiency and to inform *P. vivax* case management using primaquine, testing coverage is extremely low. Test coverage is low due to the need to prioritize newborn interventions and the complexity of currently available G6PD tests, especially those used to inform malaria case management. More affordable, accurate, point-of-care (POC) tests for G6PD deficiency are emerging that create an opportunity to extend testing to populations that do not have access to high throughput screening services. Some of these tests are quantitative, which provides an opportunity to address the gender disparity created by the currently available POC qualitative tests that misclassify females with intermediate G6PD activity as normal. In populations where the epidemiology for G6PD deficiency and *P. vivax* overlap, screening for G6PD deficiency at birth to inform care of the newborn can also be used to inform malaria case management over their lifetime.

Keywords: glucose-6-phosphate dehydrogenase; G6PD deficiency; point-of-care; diagnostics; malaria; *Plasmodium vivax*

1. Introduction

Glucose-6-phosphate dehydrogenase (G6PD) deficiency is one of the most common X-linked genetic blood disorders in the world, impacting more than 400 million people. Individuals that are G6PD deficient can develop severe jaundice in the neonatal period and acute hemolytic anemia when exposed to certain infections and drugs or when ingesting certain foods such as fava beans [1,2].

Females carry two copies of the G6PD gene, such that they can be homozygous for normal alleles ($g6pd_{norm/norm}$), homozygous for deficient alleles ($g6pd_{def/def}$) or heterozygous with one deficient and one normal G6PD allele ($g6pd_{def/norm}$). Wild-type homozygous females will present phenotypically as normal, with a G6PD activity level greater than 80% of the normal activity level, and homozygous females with two deficient alleles will present with a G6PD activity level less than 30%. However, heterozygous females with a deficient and a normal allele have a much broader phenotype, which lies mostly in the intermediate 20–80% G6PD activity ranges. With a single allele, G6PD activity levels in males are either normal or deficient [3–7].

G6PD deficiency is relevant to newborns because of the higher risk neonates with G6PD deficiency face in developing non-physiologic hyperbilirubinemia. Elevated levels of serum bilirubin (SBR) can pass the blood-brain barrier and lead to a range of neurologic disorders, including acute bilirubin-induced encephalopathy, kernicterus (chronic neurologic disease), and even death [8–10]. In term and late preterm newborns ($\geq$35 weeks of gestational age), hyperbilirubinemia can be treated with blue-light phototherapy and, in the most severe cases, with exchange transfusion following universally-accepted guidelines based on an age-specific SBR nomogram.

Severe hyperbilirubinemia usually develops within one week of birth but can also develop at a later stage. A hospital or birthing center's ability to monitor SBR levels is crucial for clinical management. In places where SBR testing is not routine, the ability to identify risk factors of hyperbilirubinemia before hospital discharge (ideally at birth) should prompt SBR testing and, together with parents and health workers, instigate education about signs of hyperbilirubinemia and guide the follow-up at home. For newborns with G6PD deficiency in particular, clinical management both in the hospital and at home includes an avoidance of hemolytic triggers (including drugs, food, and other substances). In 1989, the World Health Organization (WHO) working group on G6PD deficiency recommended that "whenever possible, neonatal screening should be performed . . . in populations where G6PD deficiency is common (i.e., where it affects more than three to five percent of males)" [11].

Geographically, G6PD deficiency is ethnically constrained, resulting in significant variability in risk, even within limited geographical boundaries [12,13]. Overall, populations with historic or current exposure to malaria typically have higher prevalence for G6PD deficiency with a mean prevalence of approximately 8.0% in malaria-endemic countries [12]. There is data to suggest that G6PD deficiency—while not protective against red blood cell invasion from parasites—is protective against severe clinical forms of malaria, which may explain the epidemiological overlap between G6PD deficiency and malaria [14–17].

In 2016, there were an estimated 8.5 million *Plasmodium* (*P.*) *vivax* cases, representing more than 35% of malaria cases outside of Africa [18]. As countries transition from malaria control to elimination, the predominant form of malaria often also transitions from *P. falciparum* to *P. vivax*; *P. vivax* accounts for 70% of malaria cases in countries with fewer than 5000 cases per year [19]. Case management of *P. vivax* (and *P. ovale*) is complicated compared to that of *P. falciparum*, due to the ability of *P. vivax* parasites to reside dormant in the liver as hypnozoites [20,21]. Hypnozoites are not susceptible to typical antimalarial drugs, which target the blood forms of the parasite, and can therefore cause relapse of the disease, weeks or months after primary infection. Relapse infections are a major source of disease burden in *P. vivax*–endemic populations [22,23]. The only class of antimalarial drugs that can cure individuals of *P. vivax* malaria is 8-aminoquinoline drugs; however, they can cause severe hemolysis in patients with G6PD deficiency. Historically, a high-dose, 14-day regimen of primaquine has been used for a radical cure of patients with *P. vivax*. Recently, tafenoquine, under the brand name of Krintafel, was approved by the Food and Drug Administration as a single-dose regimen to treat patients with confirmed *P. vivax* infection. WHO recommends testing for G6PD deficiency before administration of primaquine [24], and given the toxicity profile of the single-dose regime, testing will be required prior to administration of tafenoquine.

Due to an increased awareness of the morbidity caused by *P. vivax* relapse, the contribution of *P. vivax* relapse to onward malaria transmission, the commitment to malaria elimination in many predominantly *P. vivax*–endemic countries and the imminent availability of tafenoquine, there is renewed focus to address relapsed *P. vivax* infections by increasing access to a radical cure. In response, diagnostics manufacturers have advanced the development of point-of-care tests for G6PD deficiency that will be required for use in malaria case management.

This review discusses the overlap between screening for G6PD deficiency in newborns and testing for G6PD deficiency to inform malaria case management as well as the availability of new technologies that can bring G6PD testing to underserved and remote populations where G6PD deficiency and *P. vivax* malaria predominates.

2. Testing for G6PD Deficiency

The G6PD deficiency status of an individual can be characterized by genotype or by phenotype (Table 1). There are increasingly effective tools for G6PD genotyping both in terms of cost and timeliness [25]. For males, the genotype is sufficient to unambiguously assign a phenotype. For females, the genotype of females heterozygous for a G6PD normal and a G6PD deficient allele cannot be unambiguously phenotypically classified as their blood enzyme activities can range between 20–80% of a normal value, with the majority close to the 50% normal activity range. Regardless, it can be anticipated that G6PD genotyping will increase in screening programs through next-generation sequencing assays [26–28].

The G6PD phenotype is primarily described in terms of G6PD activity normalized for hemoglobin or red blood cell count. It has been challenging to define a single universal normal (100%) G6PD activity value, so that classification of the G6PD status of an individual is defined as the percentage of a normal value determined locally. G6PD phenotype classifications for purposes of test performance evaluation were recently described by the WHO [29]. Males with less than 30% activity are considered as deficient and males with greater than 30% activity should be considered as normal [29]. Females with less than 30%, 30–80%, and greater than 80% G6PD activity are considered G6PD deficient, intermediate, and normal, respectively [29]. Another way of defining the phenotype is by cytochemistry, wherein individual red blood cells are labeled for G6PD activity levels, and then, typically either by eye (if by microscopy) or by gating (if by flow cytometry), cells are dichotomously classified as deficient or normal and the ratio of the two can then inform a phenotypic classification (Table 1). While extremely informative, this latter approach is primarily used as a research tool and will not be further described here. From a clinical perspective, it is the G6PD phenotype that informs the risk of someone developing G6PD deficiency–related pathologies.

The biochemical assays that measure enzyme activity include two categories of G6PD tests, qualitative and quantitative. By convention, a G6PD deficient individual is considered a true positive, and a G6PD normal individual a true negative, such that sensitivity refers to the ability of a test to identify all true G6PD deficient individuals and specificity is the ability of the test to identify all true G6PD normals. A quantitative test is used as the reference standard [29,30]. The qualitative tests can only really discriminate G6PD deficient individuals from intermediate and normal individuals, and as such, heterozygous females with G6PD activity 30–40% of normal are typically classified as normal even though they have very low G6PD activity levels [30,31]. The qualitative tests have a discriminatory threshold for deficient and normal at the 30–40% activity level and can display good sensitivity for deficient males, and females with two G6PD deficient alleles, as they typically have G6PD activity below 30% normal. If there is a need to differentiate heterozygous females with low intermediate activity levels (40–50%) from G6PD normal individuals, or in other words raise the threshold G6PD activity level, the sensitivity of the qualitative test then begins to drop [31]. However, with a quantitative test, as long as there is good correlation with the reference assay, and with a gradient close to unity, the sensitivity can be kept high along the whole dynamic G6PD activity range. The most widely used qualitative test and the clinical standard of care in most hospitals is the fluorescent spot test (FST), which consists of observing nicotinamide adenine dinucleotide phosphate (NADPH) production under a long wave ultraviolet light source [32]. In newborns, the above-described limitation of the qualitative test combined with the high reticulocyte counts typically leads to a misdiagnosis of females with low G6PD activity levels at risk of developing G6PD-associated complications as normals. In other words: the sensitivity drops. There is an increasing recognition that the thresholds for defining newborns at risk of G6PD-associated complications need to be higher than the discriminatory cutoffs used by qualitative tests such as the FST [33–36].

In the context of G6PD screening, the most common approach has been to include G6PD screening within other screening programs that are typically congenital hypothyroidism screening. In these programs, the specimen source is often the heel stick (in some cases, cord blood), stored and transferred via dried blood spots (DBS), commonly known as the Guthrie card. Samples are assessed primarily via qualitative or quantitative biochemical methods, although genotyping is also performed. Screening typically utilizes high throughput instrumentation. Several strong external quality assurance systems have been put in place to assure the quality of these large volume testing facilities [37,38].

Table 1. Association between genotype and phenotype. Two methods of measuring phenotype are shown: (1) by cytochemical staining, where red blood cells (RBC) are arbitrarily assigned as having high glucose-6-phosphate dehydrogenase (G6PD) activity or low G6PD activity [5] and (2) by spectrophotometric G6PD enzyme activity measurement in whole blood. The activity is described in terms of percentage of a population's normal value [39,40].

Genotype		Phenotype	
		% RBC with High G6PD Activity (Cytometry)	% Normal G6PD Activity (Spectrophotometry)
Males			
hemizygous normal	(+)	>85%	>30%
hemizygous deficient	(−)	<10%	≤30%
Females			
homozygous normal	(+$_1$/+$_1$)	>85%	>70%
heterozygous normal	(+$_1$/+$_2$)		
heterozygous normal/deficient	(+/−)	10–85%	~20–80%
heterozygous deficient	(−$_1$/−$_2$)	<10%	≤30%
homozygous deficient	(−$_1$/−$_1$)		

3. Newborn Screening Practices for G6PD Deficiency

A recent review focusing on G6PD deficiency testing within newborn screening (NBS) practices highlights a heterogeneity in practices that are not directly correlated to the prevalence of G6PD deficiency within a country [41]. Africa and the Middle East present the highest prevalence of G6PD deficiency; however, these regions have the lowest coverage of newborn screening for G6PD deficiency. Newborn screening coverage for G6PD deficiency is the highest in the Asia Pacific region, with at least six countries providing full coverage and several also providing this service to sub-populations or access to private-sector services [41]. Additionally, in many countries that conduct newborn screening for G6PD deficiency, screening is primarily accessible to urban populations near facilities that provide the service.

Expert guidance from neonatologists has outlined key considerations when deciding whether or not to adopt or scale newborn screening for G6PD deficiency [42]. Key questions are: (1) whether testing should take place before babies leave the hospital, (2) whether screening should be universal or targeted toward babies at greatest risk and (3) what screening method should be used [43]. Additional considerations include the cost-effectiveness of screening, the frequency and severity of G6PD deficiency in a specific population, availability and efficacy of appropriate diagnostics options, and the capacity of the health system to provide appropriate counseling to parents and providers [44,45]. Sections 3.1 and 3.2 below describe practices in some countries in the context of these considerations and are by no means comprehensive.

3.1. Newborn Screening for G6PD Deficiency in the United States and Europe

In the United States, screening for G6PD deficiency is only routinely done through the newborn screening programs in two states: Pennsylvania and DC [41,46,47]. Facilities outside of those states may choose to adopt universal or targeted screening practices independently [41,47]. In Europe, newborn screening guidelines vary widely with little consensus on what should be included. Greece is the only country with nationwide coverage, while Italy has partial coverage and other countries have targeted programs [41,48]. However, in both the United States and Europe, migration makes it increasingly complicated to predict the prevalence of G6PD deficiency, the specific genotype, and the risk that certain newborn complications are related to G6PD status [49].

The American Academy of Pediatrics recommends that newborns with jaundice are screened for G6PD deficiency when family history or background suggests a likelihood of G6PD deficiency or when the response to phototherapy is poor [50–52]. Multiple methods are used for newborn screening with varying performance [53,54]. In the United States, some reports have concluded that fluorescent spot test (FST) methods are sufficient, while others indicate they are inadequate, particularly for females, due to the lack of an accurate quantitative measurement [55–58].

There is some concern that among clinicians practicing in the United States, the prevalence and clinical implications of G6PD deficiency are underappreciated [59]. Nonetheless, it is evident that American clinicians support newborn screening for G6PD [60–62]. There is some evidence to suggest that hospital-based G6PD deficiency screening is feasible and that, when paired with parental education around risk factors and triggers, the negative health impacts from hyperbilirubinemia are limited [9,47,63]. In Greece, an assessment of the national screening program from 1977–1989 was deemed justified in areas of high G6PD prevalence [64,65]. Similarly, a robust G6PD newborn screening program paired with health education programs implemented in the Sassari district of Sardinia, Italy, was associated with a 75% decline in clinical complications associated with G6PD deficiency. Notably, this decline was disproportionally observed among boys, suggesting that the intervention is less effective in girls, possibly driven by inadequacies in the screening method for female populations [66].

3.2. Newborn Screening for G6PD Deficiency in the Asia Pacific

The prevalence of G6PD deficiency is close to or more than 5% throughout the Asia Pacific region, but many countries do not have NBS programs, and for countries that do, the programs are often inefficient, with many excluding screening for G6PD deficiency. Countries of the Greater Mekong subregion where G6PD deficiency is high (Thailand, Myanmar, Laos, Vietnam and Cambodia) currently have no NBS programs despite evidence indicating a need otherwise [67].

For example, in Thailand, several studies have shown a high prevalence of G6PD deficiency [68,69] as well as an association of the deficiency with neonatal hyperbilirubinemia; however, a national NBS program for G6PD deficiency has not been set up [70–72]. Similarly, an NBS program for G6PD deficiency in Indonesia has not been implemented; a few private hospitals may screen for G6PD deficiency in newborns, while others will screen for G6PD deficiency only when there is an indication of non-physiological jaundice. While NBS in Indonesia started in 1999, it was only for congenital hypothyroidism using a heel stick sample, and coverage is <1% despite this being a national program [73], indicating a large systemic obstacle that would need to be addressed prior to G6PD deficiency screening implementation.

In the Philippines, where the prevalence of G6PD deficiency ranges from 4.5% to 25.7%, testing for G6PD deficiency is included in its newborn screening program, which is carried out within 24 h of birth; however, coverage remains low at 28% [74]. Both the Philippines and Taiwan implemented national NBS programs in 1998 and 1987, respectively. These programs utilize FST and have developed follow-up systems for G6PD-deficient individuals to receive follow-up confirmatory testing using spectrophotometry. In Taiwan, the follow-up system also includes medical care and genetic counseling [67].

Examples of successful G6PD deficiency newborn screening are Malaysia and Singapore. Malaysia has been conducting G6PD NBS since the 1970s from cord blood, and the coverage is >95% in the population and funded by the government [67]. Similarly, Singapore recognized the important role of G6PD deficiency in kernicterus and started NBS for G6PD deficiency in 1965 using cord blood as well [75]. The reported nationwide coverage for NBS is >99%. The government subsidized about 40–60% of the cost of NBS within public hospitals and has since eradicated kernicterus due to G6PD deficiency [67]. The current policy is to keep G6PD-deficient babies longer in hospitals to avoid hemolytic triggers from the environment [76].

4. G6PD Testing for Malaria Case Management

In contrast, G6PD testing to inform malaria case management using primaquine has typically not been possible due to the complexity of current G6PD test methods, which are not compatible with the remote and under-resourced clinical and laboratory settings where a majority of malaria patients seek care (Figure 1). In recent years, there has been an increase in the availability of point-of-care tests for G6PD deficiency. The CareStart G6PD (Access Bio, Somerset, NJ, USA) rapid diagnostic test is perhaps most aligned with these clinical settings, however, as a qualitative test it has some inherent limitations compared to quantitative tests (Table 2) [77–79]. The SD Biosensor STANDARD G6PD test (Suwon, Korea) represents a new point-of-care product that brings quantitative G6PD measurement normalized for hemoglobin capabilities to lower-tier clinical and laboratory settings [80]. Several other point-of-care tests for G6PD deficiency are also in development on different platforms, such as the Access Bio CareStart G6PD Biosensor (Somerset, NJ, USA) and the FINDER platform from Baebies (Durham, NC, USA) [56,81]. The benefit of the instrumented quantitative products is that they can address the inherent enzyme temperature variance through temperature correction, sustaining their accuracy and therefore utility over a broader temperature range, in contrast to the qualitative tests. More critically, just as for neonatal screening, quantitative testing is increasingly relevant for providing equal access to both males and females to both high-dose primaquine and the recently FDA- and TGA-cleared antimalarial drug tafenoquine [39]. However, there is an added level of complexity and cost to requiring an instrument to run G6PD tests in each facility where G6PD testing may be required.

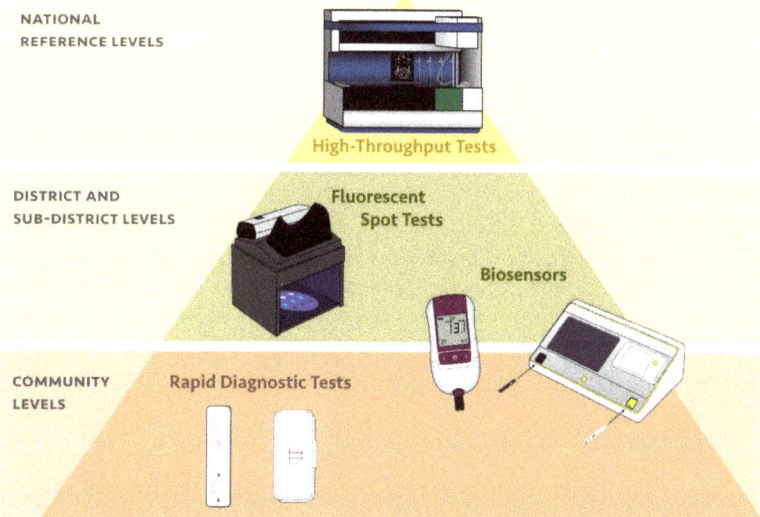

Figure 1. Alignment between diagnostic platform for G6PD deficiency and tier of health care facility based on complexity of the diagnostic test and the typical resources available at each type of facility.

Table 2. Characteristics of qualitative and quantitative point-of-care G6PD tests.

Qualitative	Quantitative
Accurately classifies males	Accurately classifies males
Females with intermediate G6PD activity classified as normal	Accurately classifies females
Does not require an instrument	Requires an instrument
Cannot correct for operating temperature, typically resulting in a more limited operating temperature range	Corrects for temperature allowing for a broader operating temperature range
Time-to-result < 10 min	Time-to-result < 10 min
Low to moderate complexity	Moderate complexity

5. New Opportunities for G6PD Screening: Synergies and Considerations

The advent of these new G6PD testing technologies raises new opportunities to address inequity in access to newborn screening in countries with high G6PD deficiency prevalence. Additionally, the overlap in epidemiology for G6PD deficiency and *P. vivax* provides a synergistic need for testing that may warrant supporting the intervention. Yet, there are several considerations that should be taken into account when assessing what technology should be included when testing is implemented.

5.1. Overlap in Desired Product Characteristics

Point-of-care G6PD tests are designed to provide fast turnaround, typically within ten minutes. This is an essential characteristic for malaria case management because patients are lost to follow-up if they are asked to return for their G6PD test result several days later. Fast turnaround is also essential for neonatal clinics in low-resource settings, as the mother and child rarely stay in the hospital longer than 24 h and systems for remote testing and test result return are highly inefficient. A limitation is that the throughput required for newborn testing is likely to be significantly higher than that for malaria testing in some settings. Additionally, the time it takes for high throughput tests to provide results may not be quick enough to inform the care of sick newborns, making a point-of-care test that can provide results within ten minutes a preferred option, even when routine screening methods are available.

5.2. Work Flow and Sample Type

The point-of-care tests that are on the market have been designed and validated for use with fresh whole blood specimens, with or without anticoagulant; however, they have not been shown to be compatible with dried blood spots, the primary specimen used in newborn screening programs. Alternatively, operations research would need to assess the feasibility of incorporating the point-of-care tests, as is, into the current workflow in delivery wards using capillary samples directly from the heel stick. In some contexts, validating the products with cord blood may be useful.

5.3. External Quality Assurance

Newborn screening programs have significantly invested in quality assurance systems, which are compatible with high throughput testing facilities but are not compatible with more decentralized lower throughput testing facilities. Quality control reagents formulated to support high throughput facilities can be amortized over many samples, which would not be the same for lower throughput facilities, resulting in significantly increasing the price of testing. Pragmatic solutions that address these differences, such as new formulations for control reagent presentation, will need to be thought out and tested.

5.4. Record Keeping

The return-on-investment or value proposition for G6PD testing at birth is highly dependent on the reliability of diagnosis done at birth and the ability of the test result to stay with the individual and individual's caretakers, which minimizes the need to retest the individual later in life. Record keeping can be very challenging in many malaria-endemic settings, which means setting- and population-specific solutions are often required.

5.5. Awareness and Sensitization

Record keeping is key for determining value proposition but is only valuable itself if the parties involved are sensitized to the implications of G6PD deficiency. This would include understanding how to prevent exposure to triggers for hyperbilirubinemia and hemolysis in G6PD-deficient individuals as well as how to identify and react according to the early onset of associated symptoms.

5.6. Cost-Effectiveness

In many low-resource settings, the priority for incorporating G6PD deficiency testing over other interventions will be hard to justify in the context of the many competing health system limitations and priorities. A series of factors will contribute to the overall value proposition in those settings, which include the prevalence of G6PD deficiency in the local population served, the likelihood that a G6PD-deficient individual will suffer associated pathologies later in life and the ability for the test result at birth to be associated with the individual throughout their life. Cost-effectiveness assessments that focus only on the short-term benefits of G6PD testing at birth are unlikely to support prioritizing the intervention. A framework for assessing the cost-effectiveness for G6PD testing at birth in settings with high prevalence of G6PD deficiency and other triggers for G6PD deficiency–associated hemolysis should be considered. These triggers can include antibiotics, certain foods, and several medications. In populations where there is also a high prevalence of *P. vivax* malaria, and radical treatment with 8-aminoquinolines is provided, the significant health benefit of preventing malaria relapse versus the costs of hospitalization of patients reacting to the drugs should be included. Cost-effectiveness models for G6PD testing for a radical cure have been developed; however, these do not integrate the use of tests at birth to avoid complications, or beyond that, of malaria case management.

6. Summary

New quantitative point-of-care technologies that address both the need for immediate results to mitigate the risk of hyperbilirubinemia and the need to provide reliable and actionable results for management of newborns or patient treatment decisions may help spur stronger and more comprehensive newborn screening efforts for G6PD deficiency in settings that do not have practical access to centralized screening programs. Testing must be accompanied with community awareness of and sensitization to G6PD deficiency along with robust record keeping such that the investments are maximized beyond the first days of life. In malaria-endemic regions, G6PD testing will provide access to the best standard of care, which is a radical cure of *P. vivax* malaria. Operations research is required to assess the feasibility and effectiveness of G6PD testing with these new point-of-care tests at birth.

Author Contributions: A.A., G.B., G.J.D., E.G.-G., S.P., A.W.S. all contributed equally to the conceptualization of the article messages, providing content, and review.

Funding: This research was funded by the Bill & Melinda Gates Foundation, grant number OPP1034534 and the UK Department for International Development (DFID), grant number 204139. The findings and conclusions contained within are those of the authors and do not necessarily reflect the positions of the Bill & Melinda Gates Foundation or the DFID.

Acknowledgments: We are grateful to Christine Waresak for proofreading the manuscript and Patrick McKern for graphics.

Conflicts of Interest: PATH supports a portfolio of G6PD test development efforts. PATH has no financial interests in the commercialization of any resulting products. The funders had no role in the design of the study; in the collection, analyses or interpretation of data; in the writing of the manuscript; and in the decision to publish the results.

References

1. Cappellini, M.D.; Fiorelli, G. Glucose-6-phosphate dehydrogenase deficiency. *Lancet* **2008**, *371*, 64–74. [CrossRef]
2. Luzzatto, L.; Nannelli, C.; Notaro, R. Glucose-6-Phosphate Dehydrogenase Deficiency. *Hematol./Oncol. Clin. N. Am.* **2016**, *30*, 373–393. [CrossRef] [PubMed]
3. Bancone, G.; Kalnoky, M.; Chu, C.S.; Chowwiwat, N.; Kahn, M.; Malleret, B.; Wilaisrisak, P.; Renia, L.; Domingo, G.J.; Nosten, F. The G6PD flow-cytometric assay is a reliable tool for diagnosis of G6PD deficiency in women and anaemic subjects. *Sci. Rep.* **2017**, *7*, 9822. [CrossRef] [PubMed]
4. Beutler, E.; Yeh, M.; Fairbanks, V.F. The normal human female as a mosaic of X-chromosome activity: Studies using the gene for C-6-PD-deficiency as a marker. *Proc. Natl. Acad. Sci. USA* **1962**, *48*, 9–16. [CrossRef] [PubMed]
5. Kalnoky, M.; Bancone, G.; Kahn, M.; Chu, C.S.; Chowwiwat, N.; Wilaisrisak, P.; Pal, S.; LaRue, N.; Leader, B.; Nosten, F.; et al. Cytochemical flow analysis of intracellular G6PD and aggregate analysis of mosaic G6PD expression. *Eur. J. Haematol.* **2018**, *100*, 294–303. [CrossRef] [PubMed]
6. Nantakomol, D.; Paul, R.; Palasuwan, A.; Day, N.P.; White, N.J.; Imwong, M. Evaluation of the phenotypic test and genetic analysis in the detection of glucose-6-phosphate dehydrogenase deficiency. *Malar. J.* **2013**, *12*, 289. [CrossRef] [PubMed]
7. Peters, A.L.; Veldthuis, M.; van Leeuwen, K.; Bossuyt, P.M.M.; Vlaar, A.P.J.; van Bruggen, R.; de Korte, D.; Van Noorden, C.J.F.; van Zwieten, R. Comparison of Spectrophotometry, Chromate Inhibition, and Cytofluorometry Versus Gene Sequencing for Detection of Heterozygously Glucose-6-Phosphate Dehydrogenase-Deficient Females. *J. Histochem. Cytochem. Off. J. Histochem. Soc.* **2017**, *65*, 627–636. [CrossRef] [PubMed]
8. Cunningham, A.D.; Hwang, S.; Mochly-Rosen, D. Glucose-6-Phosphate Dehydrogenase Deficiency and the Need for a Novel Treatment to Prevent Kernicterus. *Clin. Perinatal.* **2016**, *43*, 341–354. [CrossRef] [PubMed]
9. Kaplan, M.; Hammerman, C. Glucose-6-phosphate dehydrogenase deficiency and severe neonatal hyperbilirubinemia: A complexity of interactions between genes and environment. *Semin. Fetal Neonatal Med.* **2010**, *15*, 148–156. [CrossRef] [PubMed]
10. Olusanya, B.O.; Emokpae, A.A.; Zamora, T.G.; Slusher, T.M. Addressing the burden of neonatal hyperbilirubinaemia in countries with significant glucose-6-phosphate dehydrogenase deficiency. *Acta Paediatr.* **2014**, *103*, 1102–1109. [CrossRef] [PubMed]
11. WHO Working Group. Glucose-6-phosphate dehydrogenase deficiency. *Bull. World Health Organ.* **1989**, *67*, 601–611.
12. Howes, R.E.; Piel, F.B.; Patil, A.P.; Nyangiri, O.A.; Gething, P.W.; Dewi, M.; Hogg, M.M.; Battle, K.E.; Padilla, C.D.; Baird, J.K.; et al. G6PD deficiency prevalence and estimates of affected populations in malaria endemic countries: A geostatistical model-based map. *PLoS Med.* **2012**, *9*, e1001339. [CrossRef] [PubMed]
13. Nkhoma, E.T.; Poole, C.; Vannappagari, V.; Hall, S.A.; Beutler, E. The global prevalence of glucose-6-phosphate dehydrogenase deficiency: A systematic review and meta-analysis. *Blood Cells Mol. Dis.* **2009**, *42*, 267–278. [CrossRef] [PubMed]
14. Clarke, G.M.; Rockett, K.; Kivinen, K.; Hubbart, C.; Jeffreys, A.E.; Rowlands, K.; Jallow, M.; Conway, D.J.; Bojang, K.A.; Pinder, M.; et al. Characterisation of the opposing effects of G6PD deficiency on cerebral malaria and severe malarial anaemia. *eLife* **2017**, *6*. [CrossRef] [PubMed]
15. Ruwende, C.; Khoo, S.C.; Snow, R.W.; Yates, S.N.; Kwiatkowski, D.; Gupta, S.; Warn, P.; Allsopp, C.E.; Gilbert, S.C.; Peschu, N.; et al. Natural selection of hemi- and heterozygotes for G6PD deficiency in Africa by resistance to severe malaria. *Nature* **1995**, *376*, 246–249. [CrossRef] [PubMed]
16. Cappadoro, M.; Giribaldi, G.; O'Brien, E.; Turrini, F.; Mannu, F.; Ulliers, D.; Simula, G.; Luzzatto, L.; Arese, P. Early phagocytosis of glucose-6-phosphate dehydrogenase (G6PD)-deficient erythrocytes parasitized by Plasmodium falciparum may explain malaria protection in G6PD deficiency. *Blood* **1998**, *92*, 2527–2534. [PubMed]
17. Bancone, G.; Malleret, B.; Suwanarusk, R.; Chowwiwat, N.; Chu, C.S.; McGready, R.; Renia, L.; Nosten, F.; Russell, B. Asian G6PD-Mahidol Reticulocytes Sustain Normal Plasmodium Vivax Development. *J. Infect. Dis.* **2017**, *216*, 263–266. [CrossRef] [PubMed]
18. World Health Organization (WHO). *World Malaria Report 2017*; WHO: Geneva, Switzerland, 2017.

19. World Health Organization (WHO). *Control and Elimination of Plasmodium Vivax Malaria—A Technical Brief*; WHO: Geneva, Switzerland, 2015.
20. Baird, K.J.; Maguire, J.D.; Price, R.N. Diagnosis and treatment of Plasmodium vivax malaria. *Adv. Parasitol.* **2012**, *80*, 203–270. [CrossRef] [PubMed]
21. Chu, C.S.; White, N.J. Management of relapsing Plasmodium vivax malaria. *Expert Rev. Anti-Infect. Ther.* **2016**, *14*, 885–900. [CrossRef] [PubMed]
22. Luxemburger, C.; van Vugt, M.; Jonathan, S.; McGready, R.; Looareesuwan, S.; White, N.J.; Nosten, F. Treatment of vivax malaria on the western border of Thailand. *Trans. R. Soc. Trop. Med. Hyg.* **1999**, *93*, 433–438. [CrossRef]
23. Robinson, L.J.; Wampfler, R.; Betuela, I.; Karl, S.; White, M.T.; Li Wai Suen, C.S.; Hofmann, N.E.; Kinboro, B.; Waltmann, A.; Brewster, J.; et al. Strategies for Understanding and Reducing the Plasmodium vivax and Plasmodium ovale Hypnozoite Reservoir in Papua New Guinean Children: A Randomised Placebo-Controlled Trial and Mathematical Model. *PLoS Med.* **2015**, *12*, e1001891. [CrossRef] [PubMed]
24. World Health Organization (WHO). *Guidelines for the Treatment of Malaria*, 3rd ed.; WHO: Geneva, Switzerland, 2015.
25. Zhang, L.; Yang, Y.; Liu, R.; Li, Q.; Yang, F.; Ma, L.; Liu, H.; Chen, X.; Yang, Z.; Cui, L.; et al. A multiplex method for detection of glucose-6-phosphate dehydrogenase (G6PD) gene mutations. *Int. J. Lab. Hematol.* **2015**, *37*, 739–745. [CrossRef] [PubMed]
26. Berg, J.S.; Agrawal, P.B.; Bailey, D.B., Jr.; Beggs, A.H.; Brenner, S.E.; Brower, A.M.; Cakici, J.A.; Ceyhan-Birsoy, O.; Chan, K.; Chen, F.; et al. Newborn Sequencing in Genomic Medicine and Public Health. *Pediatrics* **2017**, *139*. [CrossRef] [PubMed]
27. Bogari, N.M. Next generation sequencing (NGS) in glucose-6-phosphate dehydrogenase (G6PD) deficiency studies. *Bioinformation* **2016**, *12*, 41–43. [CrossRef] [PubMed]
28. Holm, I.A.; Agrawal, P.B.; Ceyhan-Birsoy, O.; Christensen, K.D.; Fayer, S.; Frankel, L.A.; Genetti, C.A.; Krier, J.B.; LaMay, R.C.; Levy, H.L.; et al. The BabySeq project: Implementing genomic sequencing in newborns. *BMC Pediatr.* **2018**, *18*, 225. [CrossRef] [PubMed]
29. World Health Organization (WHO). *Technical Specifications Series for Submission to WHO Prequalification—Diagnostic Assessment: In Vitro Diagnostics Medical Devices to Identify Glucose-6-Phosphate Dehydrogenase (G6PD) Activity*; WHO: Geneva, Switzerland, 2016.
30. Domingo, G.J.; Satyagraha, A.W.; Anvikar, A.; Baird, K.; Bancone, G.; Bansil, P.; Carter, N.; Cheng, Q.; Culpepper, J.; Eziefula, C.; et al. G6PD testing in support of treatment and elimination of malaria: Recommendations for evaluation of G6PD tests. *Malar. J.* **2013**, *12*, 391. [CrossRef] [PubMed]
31. LaRue, N.; Kahn, M.; Murray, M.; Leader, B.T.; Bansil, P.; McGray, S.; Kalnoky, M.; Zhang, H.; Huang, H.; Jiang, H.; et al. Comparison of quantitative and qualitative tests for glucose-6-phosphate dehydrogenase deficiency. *Am. J. Trop. Med. Hyg.* **2014**, *91*, 854–861. [CrossRef] [PubMed]
32. Beutler, E.; Mitchell, M. Special modifications of the fluorescent screening method for glucose-6-phosphate dehydrogenase deficiency. *Blood* **1968**, *32*, 816–818. [PubMed]
33. Fu, C.; Luo, S.; Li, Q.; Xie, B.; Yang, Q.; Geng, G.; Lin, C.; Su, J.; Zhang, Y.; Wang, J.; et al. Newborn screening of glucose-6-phosphate dehydrogenase deficiency in Guangxi, China: Determination of optimal cutoff value to identify heterozygous female neonates. *Sci. Rep.* **2018**, *8*, 833. [CrossRef] [PubMed]
34. Kaplan, M.; Hammerman, C.; Vreman, H.J.; Stevenson, D.K.; Beutler, E. Acute hemolysis and severe neonatal hyperbilirubinemia in glucose-6-phosphate dehydrogenase-deficient heterozygotes. *J. Pediatr.* **2001**, *139*, 137–140. [CrossRef] [PubMed]
35. Riskin, A.; Gery, N.; Kugelman, A.; Hemo, M.; Spevak, I.; Bader, D. Glucose-6-phosphate dehydrogenase deficiency and borderline deficiency: Association with neonatal hyperbilirubinemia. *J. Pediatr.* **2012**, *161*, 191–196. [CrossRef] [PubMed]
36. Wang, F.L.; Boo, N.Y.; Ainoon, O.; Wong, M.K. Comparison of detection of glucose-6-phosphate dehydrogenase deficiency using fluorescent spot test, enzyme assay and molecular method for prediction of severe neonatal hyperbilirubinaemia. *Singap. Med. J.* **2009**, *50*, 62–67.
37. Chiang, S.H.; Wu, K.F.; Liu, T.T.; Wu, S.J.; Hsiao, K.J. Quality assurance program for neonatal screening of glucose-6-phosphate dehydrogenase deficiency. *Southeast Asian J. Trop. Med. Public Health* **2003**, *34* (Suppl. 3), 130–134. [PubMed]

38. Chiang, S.H.; Wu, S.J.; Wu, K.F.; Hsiao, K.J. Neonatal screening for glucose-6-phosphate dehydrogenase deficiency in Taiwan. *Southeast Asian J. Trop. Med. Public Health* **1999**, *30* (Suppl. 2), 72–74. [PubMed]
39. Domingo, G.J.; Advani, N.; Satyagraha, A.W.; Sibley, C.H.; Rowley, E.; Kalnoky, M.; Cohen, J.; Parker, M.; Kelley, M. Addressing the gender-knowledge gap in glucose-6-phosphate dehydrogenase deficiency: Challenges and opportunities. *Int. Health* **2018**. [CrossRef] [PubMed]
40. Chu, C.S.; Bancone, G.; Nosten, F.; White, N.J.; Luzzatto, L. Primaquine-induced haemolysis in females heterozygous for G6PD deficiency. *Malar. J.* **2018**, *17*, 101. [CrossRef] [PubMed]
41. Therrell, B.L.; Padilla, C.D.; Loeber, J.G.; Kneisser, I.; Saadallah, A.; Borrajo, G.J.; Adams, J. Current status of newborn screening worldwide: 2015. *Semin. Perinatol.* **2015**, *39*, 171–187. [CrossRef] [PubMed]
42. Leong, A. Is There a Need for Neonatal Screening of Glucose-6-Phosphate Dehydrogenase Deficiency in Canada? *McGill J. Med.* **2007**, *10*, 31–34. [PubMed]
43. Watchko, J.F.; Kaplan, M.; Stark, A.R.; Stevenson, D.K.; Bhutani, V.K. Should we screen newborns for glucose-6-phosphate dehydrogenase deficiency in the United States? *J. Perinatal. Off. J. Calif. Perinat. Assoc.* **2013**, *33*, 499–504. [CrossRef] [PubMed]
44. Nussbaum, R.; McInnes, R.; Willard, H. *Thompson & Thompson Genetics in Medicine*, 8th ed.; Elsevier/Saunders: Amsterdam, The Netherlands, 2016.
45. Watchko, J.F. Screening for glucose-6-phosphate dehydrogenase deficiency in newborns-practical considerations. *J. Pediatr.* **2012**, *161*, 179–180. [CrossRef] [PubMed]
46. Frank, J.E. Diagnosis and management of G6PD deficiency. *Am. Fam. Phys.* **2005**, *72*, 1277–1282.
47. Nock, M.L.; Johnson, E.M.; Krugman, R.R.; Di Fiore, J.M.; Fitzgerald, S.; Sandhaus, L.M.; Walsh, M.C. Implementation and analysis of a pilot in-hospital newborn screening program for glucose-6-phosphate dehydrogenase deficiency in the United States. *J. Perinatal. Off. J. Calif. Perinat. Assoc.* **2011**, *31*, 112–117. [CrossRef] [PubMed]
48. Gonzalez-Quiroga, G.; Ramirez del Rio, J.L.; Ortiz-Jalomo, R.; Garcia-Contreras, R.F.; Cerda-Flores, R.M.; Mata-Cardenas, B.D.; Garza-Chapa, R. Relative frequency of glucose-6-phosphate dehydrogenase deficiency in jaundiced newborn infants in the metropolitan area of Monterrey, Nuevo Leon. *Arch. Investig. Med.* **1990**, *21*, 223–227.
49. Manu Pereira Mdel, M.; Cabot, A.; Martinez Gonzalez, A.; Sitja Navarro, E.; Cararach, V.; Sabria, J.; Boixaderas, J.; Teixidor, R.; Bosch, A.; Lopez Vilchez, M.A.; et al. Neonatal screening of hemoglobinopathies and G6PD deficiency in Catalonia (Spain). Molecular study of sickle cell disease associated with alpha thalassemia and G6PD deficiency. *Med. Clin.* **2007**, *129*, 161–164.
50. Kaplan, M.; Hammerman, C. Severe neonatal hyperbilirubinemia. A potential complication of glucose-6-phosphate dehydrogenase deficiency. *Clin. Perinatol.* **1998**, *25*, 575–590. [CrossRef]
51. Valaes, T. Severe neonatal jaundice associated with glucose-6-phosphate dehydrogenase deficiency: Pathogenesis and global epidemiology. *Acta Paediatr.* **1994**, *394*, 58–76. [CrossRef]
52. American Academy of Pediatrics Subcommittee on Hyperbilirubinemia. Management of hyperbilirubinemia in the newborn infant 35 or more weeks of gestation. *Pediatrics* **2004**, *114*, 297–316. [CrossRef]
53. Lin, Z.; Fontaine, J.M.; Freer, D.E.; Naylor, E.W. Alternative DNA-based newborn screening for glucose-6-phosphate dehydrogenase deficiency. *Mol. Genet. Metab.* **2005**, *86*, 212–219. [CrossRef] [PubMed]
54. Reclos, G.J.; Hatzidakis, C.J.; Schulpis, K.H. Glucose-6-phosphate dehydrogenase deficiency neonatal screening: Preliminary evidence that a high percentage of partially deficient female neonates are missed during routine screening. *J. Med. Screen.* **2000**, *7*, 46–51. [CrossRef] [PubMed]
55. Lam, R.; Li, H.; Nock, M.L. Assessment of G6PD screening program in premature infants in a NICU. *J. Perinatol.* **2015**, *35*, 1027. [CrossRef] [PubMed]
56. Bhutani, V.K.; Kaplan, M.; Glader, B.; Cotten, M.; Kleinert, J.; Pamula, V. Point-of-Care Quantitative Measure of Glucose-6-Phosphate Dehydrogenase Enzyme Deficiency. *Pediatrics* **2015**, *136*, e1268–e1275. [CrossRef] [PubMed]
57. Zaffanello, M.; Rugolotto, S.; Zamboni, G.; Gaudino, R.; Tato, L. Neonatal screening for glucose-6-phosphate dehydrogenase deficiency fails to detect heterozygote females. *Eur. J. Epidemiol.* **2004**, *19*, 255–257. [CrossRef] [PubMed]
58. Stuhrman, G.; Perez Juanazo, S.J.; Crivelly, K.; Smith, J.; Andersson, H.; Morava, E. False-Positive Newborn Screen Using the Beutler Spot Assay for Galactosemia in Glucose-6-Phosphate Dehydrogenase Deficiency. *JIMD Rep.* **2017**, *36*, 1–5. [CrossRef] [PubMed]

59. Kaplan, M.; Hammerman, C. Glucose-6-phosphate dehydrogenase deficiency: A hidden risk for kernicterus. *Semin. Perinatal.* **2004**, *28*, 356–364. [CrossRef]
60. Koopmans, J.; Ross, L.F. Does familiarity breed acceptance? The influence of policy on physicians' attitudes toward newborn screening programs. *Pediatrics* **2006**, *117*, 1477–1485. [CrossRef] [PubMed]
61. Bernardo, J.; Nock, M. Pediatric Provider Insight into Newborn Screening for G6PD Deficiency. *Clin. Pediatr.* **2015**, *54*, 575–578. [CrossRef] [PubMed]
62. Christensen, R.D.; Nussenzveig, R.H.; Yaish, H.M.; Henry, E.; Eggert, L.D.; Agarwal, A.M. Causes of hemolysis in neonates with extreme hyperbilirubinemia. *J. Perinatal. Off. J. Calif. Perinat. Assoc.* **2014**, *34*, 616–619. [CrossRef] [PubMed]
63. Watchko, J.F. Hyperbilirubinemia and Bilirubin Toxicity in the Late Preterm Infant. *Clin. Perinatal.* **2006**, *33*, 839–852. [CrossRef] [PubMed]
64. Missiou-Tsagaraki, S. Screening for glucose-6-phosphate dehydrogenase deficiency as a preventive measure: Prevalence among 1,286,000 Greek newborn infants. *J. Pediatr.* **1991**, *119*, 293–299. [CrossRef]
65. Piomelli, S.; Wolff, J.A. Neonatal screening for glucose-6-phosphate dehydrogenase deficiency. *J. Pediatr.* **1992**, *121*, 497. [CrossRef]
66. Meloni, T.; Forteleoni, G.; Meloni, G.F. Marked decline of favism after neonatal glucose-6-phosphate dehydrogenase screening and health education: The northern Sardinian experience. *Acta Haematol.* **1992**, *87*, 29–31. [CrossRef] [PubMed]
67. Padilla, C.D.; Therrell, B.L. Newborn screening in the Asia Pacific region. *J. Inherit. Metab. Dis.* **2007**, *30*, 490–506. [CrossRef] [PubMed]
68. Charoenkwan, P.; Tantiprabha, W.; Sirichotiyakul, S.; Phusua, A.; Sanguansermsri, T. Prevalence and molecular characterization of glucose-6-phosphate dehydrogenase deficiency in northern Thailand. *Southeast Asian J. Trop. Med. Public Health* **2014**, *45*, 187–193. [PubMed]
69. Ratrisawadi, V.; Horpaopan, S.; Chotigeat, U.; Sangtawesin, V.; Kanjanapattanakul, W.; Ningsanond, V.; Sunthornthepvarakul, T.; Khooarmompatana, S.; Charoensiriwatana, W. Neonatal screening program in Rajavithi Hospital, Thailand. *Southeast Asian J. Trop. Med. Public Health* **1999**, *30* (Suppl. 2), 28–32.
70. Sanpavat, S.; Nuchprayoon, I.; Kittikalayawong, A.; Ungbumnet, W. The value of methemoglobin reduction test as a screening test for neonatal glucose 6-phosphate dehydrogenase deficiency. *J. Med. Assoc. Thail.* **2001**, *84* (Suppl. 1), S91–S98.
71. Tanpaichitr, V.S. Glucose-6-phosphate dehydrogenase deficiency in Thailand; its significance in the newborn. *Southeast Asian J. Trop. Med. Public Health* **1999**, *30* (Suppl. 2), 75–78.
72. Tanphaichitr, V.S.; Pung-amritt, P.; Yodthong, S.; Soongswang, J.; Mahasandana, C.; Suvatte, V. Glucose-6-phosphate dehydrogenase deficiency in the newborn: Its prevalence and relation to neonatal jaundice. *Southeast Asian J. Trop. Med. Public Health* **1995**, *26* (Suppl. 1), 137–141.
73. Rustama, D.S.; Fadil, M.R.; Harahap, E.R.; Primadi, A. Newborn screening in Indonesia. *Southeast Asian J. Trop. Med. Public Health* **2003**, *34* (Suppl. 3), 76–79.
74. Padilla, C.D. Newborn screening in the Philippines. *Southeast Asian J. Trop. Med. Public Health* **2003**, *34* (Suppl. 3), 87–88.
75. Joseph, R. Mass newborn screening in Singapore—position and projections. *Ann. Acad. Med. Singap.* **2003**, *32*, 318–323. [PubMed]
76. Care of the Newborn. Available online: https://www.healthhub.sg/live-healthy/1047/pregnancy-care-of-the-newborn (accessed on 13 September 2018).
77. Espino, F.E.; Bibit, J.A.; Sornillo, J.B.; Tan, A.; von Seidlein, L.; Ley, B. Comparison of Three Screening Test Kits for G6PD Enzyme Deficiency: Implications for Its Use in the Radical Cure of Vivax Malaria in Remote and Resource-Poor Areas in the Philippines. *PLoS ONE* **2016**, *11*, e0148172. [CrossRef] [PubMed]
78. Henriques, G.; Phommasone, K.; Tripura, R.; Peto, T.J.; Raut, S.; Snethlage, C.; Sambo, I.; Sanann, N.; Nguon, C.; Adhikari, B.; et al. Comparison of glucose-6 phosphate dehydrogenase status by fluorescent spot test and rapid diagnostic test in Lao PDR and Cambodia. *Malaria J.* **2018**, *17*, 243. [CrossRef] [PubMed]
79. Roca-Feltrer, A.; Khim, N.; Kim, S.; Chy, S.; Canier, L.; Kerleguer, A.; Tor, P.; Chuor, C.M.; Kheng, S.; Siv, S.; et al. Field trial evaluation of the performances of point-of-care tests for screening G6PD deficiency in Cambodia. *PLoS ONE* **2014**, *9*, e116143. [CrossRef] [PubMed]

80. Pal, S.; Bansil, P.; Bancone, G.; Hrutkay, S.; Kahn, M.; Gornsawun, G.; Penpitchaporn, P.; Chu, C.S.; Nosten, F.; Domingo, G.J. Evaluation of a novel quantitative test for G6PD deficiency: Bringing quantitative testing for G6PD deficiency closer to the patient. *Am. J. Trop. Med.* **2018**. [CrossRef] [PubMed]
81. Bancone, G.; Gornsawun, G.; Chu, C.S.; Porn, P.; Pal, S.; Bansil, P.; Domingo, G.J.; Nosten, F. Validation of the quantitative point-of-care CareStart biosensor for assessment of G6PD activity in venous blood. *PLoS ONE* **2018**, *13*, e0196716. [CrossRef] [PubMed]

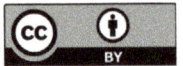
© 2018 by the authors. Licensee MDPI, Basel, Switzerland. This article is an open access article distributed under the terms and conditions of the Creative Commons Attribution (CC BY) license (http://creativecommons.org/licenses/by/4.0/).

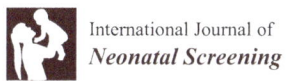

Review

Improving Screening Programmes for Sickle Cell Disorders and Other Haemoglobinopathies in Europe: The Role of Patient Organisations

John James * and Elizabeth Dormandy

Sickle Cell Society, London NW10 4UA, UK; elizabethdormandy@gmail.com
* Correspondence: john.james@sicklecellsociety.org

Received: 31 December 2018; Accepted: 25 January 2019; Published: 29 January 2019

Abstract: This discussion paper has been written to show the unique contribution and added value that Patient Organisations can give to the development and improvement of newborn screening programmes for sickle cell disorder (SCD) and other haemoglobinopathies in Europe. As an example, the action of the Sickle Cell Society (SCS) in partnership with statutory organisations in the U.K., such as the National Health Service (NHS) Sickle Cell and Thalassaemia Screening Programme (NHS SCT SP), will be described.

Keywords: sickle cell disorder; patient organisations; patient representatives; service users; sickle cell and thalassaemia screening programme; health policy

1. Background

Sickle cell disorders and thalassaemias are severe genetic disorders impairing haemoglobin function and/or production of the red blood cells. Both result in a significant morbidity and an increased risk of mortality, starting in the first years of life. Sickle cell disorder (SCD) has become the most common genetic disorder in several countries in Europe, most notably in France and the U.K., with overall prevalences of 1/1836 and 1/2439 newborns, respectively, in 2016 [1,2]. In Europe, only France, the U.K., the Netherlands and Spain have national newborn screening programmes for SCD. In the U.K., newborn screening has been set up in England and Scotland, and Wales and Northern Ireland have by and large followed the policy set in England. All these national programmes offer universal screening with the exception of France where a targeted programme is offered only to at-risk couples. Belgium has two regional programmes (Brussels and Liège) and there are pilot programmes in Italy, Germany and Ireland. Following migration and demographic changes there are an increasing number of people at risk of haemoglobinopathies in Europe, particularly in Germany and Italy. It has been noted that extension of the newborn screening is badly needed [3]. Recently, a consensus statement and recommendation for screening programmes has been produced [4].

Newborn screening programmes, with early implementation of comprehensive follow-up and prevention of the major complications, have dramatically improved survival in children with SCD in the U.S., the U.K. and France [5–7].

In the U.K., the NHS SCT Screening Programme is a linked antenatal and newborn screening programme. It uses the Family Origin Questionnaire and blood tests to screen pregnant women (and the baby's biological father, where relevant) to identify those at risk of having a baby with either one or two serious inherited blood disorders—SCD and thalassaemia major. It also screens all newborn babies for SCD, as part of the newborn blood spot programme. Antenatal screening aims to offer pregnant women and their families reproductive choice. Newborn screening aims to identify affected babies, so that they can enter care and receive appropriate treatment before they become unwell. This can improve not only the quality of life of babies but also that of their parents/family. In the five-year period of 2010–2015, 1317 babies with sickle cell disease were identified in England [8]. In 2016/2017 677,000 pregnant women were screened and 667,500 newborn babies were screened [2].

The introduction of the NHS Sickle Cell and Thalassaemia Screening Programme in England has been the major driving force for improvements both in awareness and in the quality of care for children with SCD and other major haemoglobinopathies [9].

2. Role of the Patient Organisations

As a patient organisation, the Sickle Cell Society (SCS) works closely with people living with sickle cell, their families, NHS bodies (commissioners and providers), Government, Pharma Industry and a range of other national stakeholders and voluntary sector organisations.

Since the inception of the Screening Programme in 2001, the SCS has worked in partnership with the NHS Sickle Cell and Thalassaemia Programme and has been flexible in dealing with organisational changes within the NHS. The focus of that work has consistently been outreach work. For example, to address ignorance and stigma about SCD, the SCS has engaged with communities less likely to access health information through usual NHS channels, particularly men. The SCS produced a DVD entitled The Family Legacy to educate and improve knowledge about SCD in African communities [10]. Literature for families at risk has been produced jointly by the SCS and the Screening Programme, resulting in information that meets the needs of families with SCD [11,12]. The SCS has also acted as a bridge between health services and service users in the development of a National Haemoglobinopathy Register, resulting in a register that has ownership by service users. This in part is evidenced by the continuing increase of people living with SCD being registered on the National Haemoglobinopathy Register. As well as outreach work, the SCS has worked with the NHS SCT SP to influence policy through an All Party Parliamentary Group, Chaired by Diane Abbott MP [13].

The SCS has also worked with the NHS SCT SP and other organisations in developing and monitoring standards for the care of children and adults with SCD [14]. This work showed that 99% of screen positive babies were referred to a designated healthcare professional by 8 weeks of age and 85% of screen positive babies are seen in specialist treatment centres by 3 months [8]. The monitoring of these standards was a joint project between the SCS, U.K. Thalassaemia Society (UKTS) and NHS SCT SP. This joint collaboration ensured that patients had a say in how their data was being used. Ethical approval for the data collection specifically mentioned how important the engagement of the voluntary sector was in granting ethical approval. It is not possible to determine if the collaboration has led to increased diagnoses.

Now that the Screening Programme is well established, the focus has been on improving the screening pathway for pregnant women and their families. In March 2015, the SCS, UKTS and NHS SCT SP set up a small group of parents of children with SCD and thalassaemia together with health professionals from disciplines including obstetric, genetics and midwifery. The work of the group focussed on understanding and identifying the causes for why women with these conditions are tested late. The SCS in partnership with UKTS were commissioned to do this work on behalf of the NHS SCT SP [15]. As a direct result of the work of SCS and U.K. Thalassaemia Society and the lessons learned from the experiences of parents, the Screening Programme was able to update its standards and guidelines and public and professional educational resources. For example, an improved service pathway for at-risk couples was put in place by the Screening Programme. One of the most important lessons from this work was to bust the myth that late testing is due to late presentation by women. The majority of women first presented in pregnancy at less than 10 weeks of gestation and already knew they were carriers of the sickle cell or thalassaemia gene [15]. Collaborative working with the SCS and UKTS has been beneficial both for service users and health care professionals—it provides service users with a stronger voice and reduces the need for healthcare professionals to work with different service user groups. Other collaborations between patient organisations have been established, such as the Thalassaemia International Federation (TIF). One advantage for the Sickle Cell Society and the UKTS is the ability to work with one screening programme.

The SCS as a patient-led organisation provides expertise derived from work with patients/families on peer support, research and development, advocacy, education and policy development, as well as an independent patient perspective. This assists the NHS SCTP in gaining a better understanding of the patient/family perspective. It also assists them in assessing screening policy developments and the potential impact on the experience of service users.

Underlying this partnership approach is a recognition by the SCS that SCD is an underserved condition in the U.K., Europe and beyond, when compared to like inherited conditions such as Cystic Fibrosis. Our partnership is also focussed on addressing those inequities and reducing health inequalities.

3. Issues and Challenges

The austerity and financial challenges that face the NHS in the U.K., such as rising demand and a growing elderly population, place an increased burden on patient organisations such as the SCS to mobilise, advocate and empower patients/families to educate and work even more closely with external organisations such as the NHS Sickle Cell and Screening Programme.

Over the past five years, the SCS has changed significantly, and it continues to evolve. This change and evolution has been positive both internally and with external stakeholders such as the NHS SCT Screening Programme. In particular, we have enhanced our credibility and built strong relationships with our external Screening Programme colleagues. This is important because patient organisations have to continually demonstrate their credibility and professionalism without compromising their representativeness. This, in part, is evidenced by the SCS's ability to secure a two-year tender from the Screening Programme between April 2016 and July 2018 to continue targeted outreach work. The SCS and UKTS have since been successful in bidding for a two-year extension to this work. Lack of funding and resources is a constant challenge, so contracts awarded by the public sector that extend beyond one year are particularly valuable to patient organisations.

4. Conclusions

The role played by the Sickle Cell Society as a Patient Organisation is constantly evolving in an ever-changing NHS landscape, which requires from us credibility, professionalism and the ability to deliver programmes of work supporting public sector organisations. Our partnership work with the Screening Programme is based on our core principles of representing the voice of SCD patients and families, but also based on openness, transparency, collaboration and equity.

Our outreach work with the Screening Programme over the past 18 years has not only helped raise awareness of the screening pathway for patients and health professionals but it has positively influenced the policies, guidelines and educational materials of the Screening Programme. This enables services that are better placed to meet service user needs and the programme objectives. It may be possible to extend this work by strengthening links between Patient Organisations in Europe.

The Sickle Cell Society believes strongly in working in partnership with statutory and non-statutory organisations as well as directly with people living with SCD and their families. This approach of partnership has delivered positive results for partners and service users in the U.K. We believe that there is potential to develop the role of Patient Organisations across Europe to work more collaboratively with the common purpose of improving health policy for people living with SCD in Europe. This approach is in place for other conditions such as thalassaemia through the Thalassamaemia International Federation (TIF). So why not for SCD? Given the rising prevalence of SCD in Europe and the inconsistent EU-wide models of care for SCD, collaborative working between Patient Organisations will become more important.

Funding: This research received no external funding.

Conflicts of Interest: John James is employed by the Sickle Cell Society and Elizabeth Dormandy is a volunteer with the Sickle Cell Society. The authors declare no other conflict of interest.

References

1. Association Française pour le Dépistage et la Prévention des Handicaps de l'Enfant, Bilan d'activité 2016. Available online: http://www.afdphe.org/sites/default/files/bilan_afdphe_2016.pdf (accessed on 26 January 2019).
2. NHS Sickle Cell and Thalassaemia Screening Programme. Data report 2016 to 2017: Trends and Performance Analysis. Available online: https://assets.publishing.service.gov.uk/government/uploads/system/uploads/attachment_data/file/713120/SCT_data_report_2016_to_2017.pdf (accessed on 26 January 2019).
3. Shook, L.M.; Ware, R.E. Sickle cell screening in Europe: The time has come. *Br. J. Haematol.* **2018**, *183*, 534–535. [CrossRef] [PubMed]
4. Lobitz, S.; Telfer, P.; Cela, E.; Allaf, B.; Angastiniottis, M.; Backman Johansson, C.; Badens, C.; Bento, C.; Bouva, M.J.; Canatan, D.; et al. Newborn screening for sickle cell disease in Europe: Recommendations from a Pan-European Consensus Conference. *Br. J. Haematol.* **2018**, *183*, 648–660. [CrossRef] [PubMed]
5. Vichinsky, E.; Hurst, D.; Earles, A.; Kleman, K.; Lubin, B. Newborn screening for sickle cell disease: Effect on mortality. *Pediatrics* **1988**, *81*, 749–755. [PubMed]
6. Telfer, P.; Coen, P.; Chakravorty, S.; Wilkey, O.; Evans, J.; Newell, H.; Smalling, B.; Amos, R.; Stephens, A.; Rogers, D.; et al. Clinical outcomes in children with sickle cell disease living in England: A neonatal cohort in East London. *Haematologica* **2007**, *92*, 905–912. [CrossRef] [PubMed]
7. Couque, N.; Girard, D.; Ducrocq, R.; Boizeau, P.; Haouari, Z.; Missud, F.; Holvoet, L.; Ithier, G.; Belloy, M.; Odièvre, M.H.; et al. Improvement of medical care in a cohort of newborns with sickle-cell disease in North Paris: Impact of national guidelines. *Br. J. Haematol.* **2016**, *173*, 927–937. [CrossRef] [PubMed]
8. Streetly, A.; Sisodia, R.; Dick, M.; Latinovic, R.; Hounsell, K.; Dormandy, E. Evaluation of newborn sickle cell screening programme in England: 2010–2016. *Arch. Dis. Child.* **2018**, *103*, 648–653. [CrossRef] [PubMed]
9. Catherine Coppinger. Available online: https://phescreening.blog.gov.uk/2016/09/01/weve-helped-thousands-of-babies-during-10-years-of-newborn-screening-for-sickle-cell-disease/ (accessed on 26 January 2019).
10. Film: The Family Legacy. Available online: https://www.sicklecellsociety.org/resource/the-family-legacy/ (accessed on 26 January 2019).
11. Sickle Cell Society: Resources. Available online: https://www.sicklecellsociety.org/resources/ (accessed on 29 January 2019).
12. Sickle Cell Disease: Description in Brief. Available online: https://www.gov.uk/government/publications/sickle-cell-disease-description-in-brief (accessed on 28 January 2019).
13. All-Party Parliamentary Group on Sickle Cell and Thalassaemia. Available online: https://publications.parliament.uk/pa/cm/cmallparty/register/sickle-cell-and-thalassaemia.htm (accessed on 26 January 2019).
14. Standards for Clinical Care of Adults with Sickle Cell Disease in the UK-2018. Available online: https://www.sicklecellsociety.org/resource/sicklecellstandards/ (accessed on 26 January 2019).
15. Parents' Stories. Available online: https://www.sicklecellsociety.org/resource/parents-stories/ (accessed on 26 January 2019).

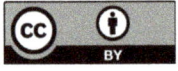

© 2019 by the authors. Licensee MDPI, Basel, Switzerland. This article is an open access article distributed under the terms and conditions of the Creative Commons Attribution (CC BY) license (http://creativecommons.org/licenses/by/4.0/).

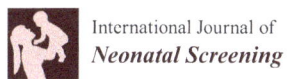

Article

Utilising the 'Getting to Outcomes®' Framework in Community Engagement for Development and Implementation of Sickle Cell Disease Newborn Screening in Kaduna State, Nigeria

Baba P.D. Inusa [1,*], Kofi A. Anie [2], Andrea Lamont [3], Livingstone G. Dogara [4], Bola Ojo [5], Ifeoma Ijei [4], Wale Atoyebi [6], Larai Gwani [7], Esther Gani [8] and Lewis Hsu [9]

1. Department Evelina Children's Hospital, Guy's and St Thomas' NHS Foundation Trust, London SE1 7EH, UK
2. Department of Haematology and Sickle Cell Centre, London North West University Healthcare NHS Trust and Imperial College, London NW10 7NS, UK; kofi.anie@nhs.net
3. Department of Implementation Science, University of South Carolina, Columbia, SC 29208, USA; alamont082@gmail.com
4. Department of Haematology, School of Medicine, Kaduna State University, Barau Dikko Teaching Hospital, Kaduna 800212, Nigeria; dogaralivingstone@gmail.com (L.G.D.); ijeiip@yahoo.com (I.I.)
5. Sickle Cell Cohort Research Foundation, WUSE Zone II, Abuja 70032, Nigeria; bolaibilola@yahoo.co.uk
6. Department of Haematology, Oxford University Hospitals NHS Foundation Trust, Oxford OX3 9DU, UK; Wale.Atoyebi@ouh.nhs.uk
7. Kaduna State Assembly Office, Kaduna 800212, Nigeria; laraigwani@gmail.com
8. Library Department, Kaduna State University, Kaduna 800241, Nigeria; ganiestty@gmail.com
9. Department of Pediatric Hematology-Oncology, University of Illinois at Chicago, Chicago, IL 60612, USA; LewHsu@UIC.EDU
* Correspondence: baba.inusa@nhs.net; Tel.: +44-20-7188-4676

Received: 8 October 2018; Accepted: 11 November 2018; Published: 16 November 2018

Abstract: Background: Sickle Cell Disease (SCD) has been designated by WHO as a public health problem in sub-Saharan Africa, and the development of newborn screening (NBS) is crucial to the reduction of high SCD morbidity and mortality. Strategies from the field of implementation science can be useful for supporting the translation of NBS evidence from high income countries to the unique cultural context of sub-Saharan Africa. One such strategy is community engagement at all levels of the healthcare system, and a widely-used implementation science framework, "Getting to Outcomes®" (GTO), which incorporates continuous multilevel evaluation by stakeholders about the quality of the implementation. Objectives: (1) to obtain critical information on potential barriers to NBS in the disparate ethnic groups and settings (rural and urban) in the healthcare system of Kaduna State in Nigeria; and, (2) to assist in the readiness assessment of Kaduna in the implementation of a sustainable NBS programme for SCD. Methods: Needs assessment was conducted with stakeholder focus groups for two days in Kaduna state, Nigeria, in November 2017. Results: The two-day focus group workshop had a total of 52 participants. Asking and answering the 10 GTO accountability questions provided a structured format to understand strengths and weaknesses in implementation. For example, we found a major communication gap between policy-makers and user groups. Conclusion: In a two-day community engagement workshop, stakeholders worked successfully together to address SCD issues, to engage with each other, to share knowledge, and to prepare to build NBS for SCD in the existing healthcare system.

Keywords: Sickle Cell Disease; 'Getting to Outcomes'; newborn screening; sub-Saharan Africa; Nigeria; Kaduna State; implementation science; public health engagement

1. Introduction

Sickle Cell Disease (SCD) has been designated by the World Health Organisation (WHO) as a public health problem in sub-Saharan Africa [1–3]. It is projected that, unless specific action is taken, the burden of disease will continue to increase into 2050, especially in Nigeria and Democratic Republic of Congo, where this increase is estimated to be more than 100% [4]. The number of annual births with SCD is estimated to be 100,000 to 150,000 in Nigeria. Our pilot Newborn screening (NBS) study of infants up to six months old in an area within Kaduna State, Nigeria, reported an incidence of 1.7% [4,5], which suggests that over 4000 babies with SCD are born every year (based on 240,000 annual overall births per state). Consistent with WHO's call to action, national and regional policies for the management and control of SCD are required, especially in the view of limited resources across most of sub-Saharan Africa. SCD represents an urgent health burden, both in terms of mortality and morbidity. It is estimated that it accounts for 8–16% of under-five mortality in sub-Saharan Africa [6]. Mortality among children with SCD in Africa is estimated at 50% to 90% by 10 years of age, mostly from preventable infections [2].

Effective management of SCD should incorporate NBS with the prevention of infections (including pneumococcal septicaemia and malaria), parental education, and support at all levels of healthcare provision to enable the timely recognition of SCD complications and health maintenance. The development of NBS programmes in sub-Saharan Africa is crucial to the reduction of high infant mortality. These programmes must be guided by empirical evidence, often accumulated in high income countries, such as United States of America (USA) and United Kingdom (UK), and simultaneously fit within the unique cultural context of sub-Saharan Africa (which is very distinct from the setting of the original clinical trial). This often poses a challenge in implementation where the original trial does not fit with the local context. Strategies from the field of implementation science, defined as the "scientific study of methods to promote the systematic uptake of research findings and other evidence-based practices into routine practice, and, hence, to improve the quality and effectiveness of health services and care" [7] can be useful for supporting the translation of evidence from clinical trials to implementation in contexts vastly different from that originally employed in the clinical trial, such as Kaduna State in Africa. One such strategy is community engagement at all levels of the healthcare system [8].

Kaduna State in northern Nigeria was the country's old colonial capital, it is a microcosm of the entire country, and has a population of over eight million made up of over 60 different ethnic groups, with 23 local governments, three geopolitical (senatorial) zones, with over 30 health care facilities for secondary care, two academic institutions (tertiary care and undergraduate training), and five teaching hospitals (tertiary care) hospitals. The academic institutions are Ahmadu Bello University Teaching Hospital and Barau Dikko Teaching Hospital, Kaduna State University, and the other four tertiary care level hospitals are National Eye Centre, National Ear Care Centre, Federal Neuro-Psychiatric Hospital, and 44 Nigerian Armed Forces Reference Hospital. The State offers free healthcare for pregnant women and children up to five years of age. Kaduna State Primary Health Care Agency is led by an Executive Secretary to oversee primary care centres and clinics in conjunction with the local governments.

We embarked on community engagement as the initial step to informing the development and implementation of an NBS programme for SCD in Kaduna State. Community engagement has been broadly defined as involving communities in information giving, consultation, decision-making, planning, co-design, governance, and delivery of services [9]. This was an early phase of sustained engagement with a broad range of community representatives to be inclusive and aimed for equal partnership. Furthermore, the application of implementation science within health systems is of benefit to the development and implementation of health interventions. Despite favourable evidence in clinical trials, programmes often fail to reach their desired outcomes in the real world due to limitations outside the trial environment and challenges with implementation.

Implementation science provides strategies to help guide implementation, therefore improving access to evidence-based services that fit with the culture of the population in need. The first phase usually consists of descriptive, formative research to better understand the major implementation challenges and to design potential strategies to overcome these [10]. We employed a widely-used implementation science framework, "Getting to Outcomes®" (GTO), which incorporates continuous multilevel evaluation by stakeholders about the quality of the implementation [11–13]. GTO is a 10-step system of accountability that guides the user through the process of planning, monitoring, and evaluating programmes. The continuous evaluation facilitates adaptation of the programme to local capacity and motivation for change, which maximizes the chances of programme success.

The objectives of the community engagement were two-fold. First, to obtain critical information pertaining to disparate ethnic groups and settings (rural and urban), including potential barriers to a successful NBS with the Kaduna State healthcare system and subsequent policy implementation. Second, to assist in the readiness assessment of Kaduna State in the implementation of a sustainable NBS programme for SCD.

2. Methods

Qualitative research methodology was employed in a two-day focus group workshop with an identical format over the two days in Kaduna. A representative group of participants were invited for each of the two focus group sessions. These comprised parents of children with SCD, adults with SCD, representatives of patient association and support groups, community leaders, health professionals, and policy-makers from the three health zones in Kaduna state, including nurses and midwives. Community health extensions workers from primary healthcare centres, doctors, and nurses from general and teaching hospitals were among the participants. In addition, five participants from the neighbouring Niger State were invited to the first focus group session to highlight the anticipated differences between states.

Focus group discussions were facilitated by a faculty of five international and local experts in SCD from the UK and Nigeria, including paediatricians, haematologists, a psychologist, and a professional in community engagement. The focus group format included brief introductory lectures on SCD and NBS. This was followed by a series of 10 questions based on the ten-point GTO framework for discussion. Each participant was given the opportunity and was encouraged to be candid with their responses and discussions in a relaxed and open atmosphere and speak in any language of their preference. Proceedings were transcribed by a professional scribe and audio-recorded. Subsequently, transcripts were produced from the audio recordings by two professionals that were experienced in transcribing (LG) and qualitative research (EG). Their combined report was reviewed by the facilitators of focus groups for accuracy and consistency (KAA, BO, and BI).

3. Results

There was a total of 52 participants for the two-day focus group workshop (Table 1). Discussions based on the GTO questions and additional issues are summarised by themes generated below.

Table 1. Participants of the Two-Day Community Engagement Focus Group Sessions.

Institution or Participant	Number
Adult with Sickle Cell Disease	2
Ahmadu Bello University Teaching Hospital–Zaria	4
Ahmadu Bello University Teaching Hospital School of Nursing–Zaria	1
Barau Dikko Teaching Hospital–Kaduna	8
Fantsuam Foundation–Kafanchan	3
Gambo Sawaba Memorial Hospital–Zaria	1
Federal Ministry of Finance–Abuja (Independent Participant)	1
Kaduna State Primary Healthcare Development Agency	2
Media Representatives	2
Mil-Goma Community Leaders–Zazzau Emirate	2
Niger State Government–(Jumai Babangida Aliyu Maternal and Neonatal Hospital) Minna, Niger State	5
Panaf Schools–Kaduna	2

Table 1. Cont.

Institution or Participant	Number
Parent of a Child/Children with Sickle Cell Disease	3
Rahma Integrated Sickle Cell Research Centre–Kaduna	1
Safiya Sickle Cell Foundation Zaria–Kaduna and Abuja	3
Samira Sanusi Sickle Cell Foundation–Kaduna	4
Sickle Cell Health Promotion Centre–Kaduna	2
Sir Patrick Ibrahim Yakowa Hospital–Kafanchan	4
Kaduna State House of Assembly	1
Kaduna State Ministry of Health and Human Services	1

3.1. Objectives of a SCD Programme

- Early detection and reduction of SCD in our communities
- To offer subsidised testing and treatment
- To minimize the cost of treatment and maintenance
- Reduce psychological and emotional trauma amongst family members
- To reduce the financial drain on the families of SCD patients
- Increase awareness of SCD most especially in the rural areas
- Improve the health status of SCD patients
- Eradicate stigma
- Healthy communities to function better
- Accurate data to inform policy makers in improved planning
- Give hope to patients with SCD to live normal fulfilled lives
- Improve standard of diagnosis to rule out confusion
- Increase the life expectancy of patients and eradication of SCD
- Reduce morbidity and mortality

3.2. Perceptions about NBS

- Early diagnosis and administering Penicillin improve on the patient's life expectancy
- Strong perception about SCD not having a cure affects the minds of families
- Poverty and financial constraint hinder families from accessing NBS
- Myths and traditional beliefs about SCD being associated with witchcraft creates an obstacle to NBS
- Most SCD babies not tested at birth end up dying from malaria even before SCD is detected

3.3. Implementation of NBS

- The early diagnosis should be at primary, secondary and tertiary health care centres
- Parents of affected children should be confidentially informed of the implication of SCD and how to prepare for the child's welfare
- World Sickle Cell Day should be emphasised with adequate publicity
- Screening, diagnosis, counselling and service delivery should be inter faced
- Blood samples should be taken at birth and in post-natal clinics
- Incentivising the process by giving out souvenirs
- NBS should be free and patients be given free or subsidized medication
- The Government should give SCD a priority

3.4. Why We Need a NBS Programme

- To create the opportunity for effective management of SCD

- To inform the community on the importance of screening
- To inform parents on how to prepare for the child's welfare
- Early detection will make the government have up to date data on SCD for adequate planning
- To increase the chances of controlling the disease
- To help in reducing stigma and disabuse the perception of the community
- To properly manage patients and parents

3.5. Best Practices to Adopt

- Community based approach by involving Volunteer Community Mobilisers (VCMs) and Traditional Birth Attendants (TBAs)
- Facility based approach
- Utilising media to disseminate information through drama on radio and television
- Incorporate the importance of NBS during antenatal health talks
- Involve community and religious organizations for sensitization campaigns like in the case of the "child spacing" campaigns
- Development partners, NGOs and media collaboration to expand
- More Sickle cell centres should be made available, accessible and affordable
- Social networks should be utilized for campaigns of SCD
- Train existing staff and employ additional qualified staff to run the centres
- Compulsory routine testing at birth
- Build linkages between the community and health care facilities

3.6. Resources and Capacity Building Needed

- Train TBAs to use simple testing for NBS
- Train Village Community Mobilisers
- Train existing staff and employ additional qualified professionals
- Existing health facilities should be equipped
- Build on existing HIV infrastructure
- Technical and financial support from development partners, and charitable organizations
- Continuous advocacy for dissemination of the facts about SCD
- Newborn testing should be available, accessible and affordable

3.7. How to Evaluate the Success of the Programme

- Using existing data to plan
- Correct and appropriate documentation is essential for evaluation
- Continuous monitoring of the programme
- Training and re-training of personnel

In addition, core themes identified within the GTO framework and categorised by the type of participant or institution are presented in Table 2.

Table 2. Ten Steps of the "Getting to Outcomes®" Framework for Sickle Cell Disease New Born Screening and Key Messages from Participants.

	Parent of Sickle Cell Disease (SCD) Child	Community Health Worker	Health Centre Doctor	Health System Hospital Administrator	Laboratory Technician	Patient Organisation Representative
Step 1: Needs & Resources	Early diagnosis & pre-marital counselling	Early awareness of SCD status	Early diagnosis & lack of treatment facilities	Innovative utilisation of resources	Equipment, reagents & quality assurance	Use of media for public awareness
Step 2: Goals & Objectives	Knowledge of diagnosis and access to treatment	Address ignorance, stigma & beliefs	Early detection of SCD and provision of medical care	Equity on service provision for SCD similar to HIV	To eliminate errors in diagnosis	Public perception about SCD
Step 3: Best Practices	Immunisation programme which is accessible	Strong educational elements of family planning campaign	HIV/AIDS programme structure & funding	Low cost intervention that is affordable	Reduce false positives & false negatives results	SCD education for families & general public
Step 4: Programme Fit for NBS	Testing during other clinics such as immunisation	Community worker leadership important	Primary health care system to reach local communities	Combine with other dried blood sample testing	Staff trained for IEF [a] & would like skills in HPLC [b] in addition	Encourage community participation
Step 5: Capacity for NBS	Staff must be competent	Partnership with community	Shortages of staff, medicines & development of skills	Limited resources, 3 tiers of government & community participation	Reagents supply, storage & inventory	Public engagement and sensitisation
Step 6: NBS Implementation Plan	Provide medicines & access to staff	Counselling, treatment for patients & families	Health status, treatment, tracking & follow up	Need to know SCD burden, resource implication	Clear standard operating procedures	Address myths & stigma
Step 7: Evaluation for NBS	Is my baby growing well?	Reporting outcome of babies visiting the SCD centre, verbal autopsies	Diagnosed babies receiving penicillin & attending SCD clinic	Infant & childhood mortality, immunisation coverage	Monthly & quarterly arranged Quality Assurance	Parliamentary oversight & reports to constituents.
Step 8: NBS Outcome Evaluation	Knowledgeable staff & a Sickle Cell Centre	Number of patients accessing counselling services	Percentage of diagnosed babies with SCD, penicillin prophylaxis	Survival for SCD children at 1, 5 & 10 years of age	Accurate & timeliness of laboratory results	A sickle cell centre for Kaduna state
Step 9: Continuous Quality Improvement	Parent support & input in care	Education & step-down training	Teleconference discussion on NBS programme results & troubleshooting	Continuous assessment & Peer Review Systems	Weekly quality reports on results, timeliness & errors	Sensitise general public, religious & community leaders
Step 10: Sustainability of NBS Programme	Not limited to a state governor's term in office	Involve all sectors of health care	Multidisciplinary team, government support	Involvement of all parties	Train personnel for additional laboratory procedures	Educate to accept responsibility of both men & women

[a] Isoelectric Focusing (IEF). [b] High Performance Liquid Chromatography (HPLC).

4. Discussion

Readiness is part of GTO, but what we did in this focus group was broader than readiness alone. We organized the findings by GTO steps, which served to (1) understand differences in perspectives across the different levels (this is important for addressing potential barriers) and (2) to remain accountable for implementation. From an implementation standpoint, one of the challenges faced in health care settings is the transport of interventions from a research trial to naturalistic setting. There are many factors that get in the way of successful implementation in naturalistic settings, especially in complex settings, like the multilevel healthcare structure in Kaduna. Differences in the vision, needs, resources, and goals of different levels of the health system may get in the way of successful implementation. This complexity is compounded by differences in contextual factors between the setting of the original clinical trial of the intervention and the local context where the intervention is being implemented. Most likely adaptations are needed to achieve the similar outcomes of a well-funded clinical trial in a developing country. In order to identify which adaptations are needed, and at which level these adaptations are needed, community engagement at each healthcare level is needed.

SCD poses a major public health problem in Nigeria. Community engagement as a first step to developing and implementing a sustainable NBS programme was carried out by SCD experts from UK, USA, and Nigeria, working with a charity in Nigeria called the Sickle Cell Cohort Research (SCORE) Foundation. Focus group discussions employing an implementation science approach with patients, parents, community leaders, doctors, nurses, and community health workers allowed active participation and important information to be gathered about the difficulties and solutions for testing newborn babies in these communities, including cultural and religious beliefs.

This study employed a well-known implementation framework to guide community engagement. Through focus groups, we uncovered certain areas where potential barriers to implementation may exist and where certain adaptations may be needed to improve the chances of achieving programmatic success. For example, we found a major communication gap between policy-makers and user groups. There is an absence of patient-users consultation within the state policy framework and therefore the lack of opportunity to incorporate their views in service planning and implementation. Asking and answering the 10 GTO accountability questions provided a structured format to understand the strengths and weaknesses in the implementation setting. This led nicely to the development of plans that support quality implementation. In this way, the hospitals will be more prepared for implementation and increase their chances of programmatic success.

The goals and objectives were addressed. Outcomes include the opportunity for participants working together to address SCD issues, to network, and engage with each other. Shared knowledge by participants, greater awareness of what is in place albeit on a small scale. Some myths and misinformation were addressed. There is no doubt that the importance of NBS for SCD programme development and implementation in Kaduna State, Niger State and the entire country cannot be over emphasised. To ensure the sustainability of the programme, the government has to be fully committed to it by providing the legal framework, policies, and adequate funding. It is also important to note that issues such as lack of public awareness and concerns could be barriers to a successful programme. Therefore, it is necessary to educate the general public through media campaigns, and advocate in partnership with the support of religious and traditional leaders within.

5. Summary and Conclusions

The two-day workshop successfully set the stage for the development and implementation plan of the NBS programme for SCD communities. Recommendations for the next steps to developing a Kaduna State NBS for SCD programme were made to the State's Commissioner of Health, and subsequently an initial four-day training workshop was organised prior to step by step implementation: (i) Procurement of reagents (ii) collection of blood spots from one local government area (1/23) of the state to test robustness of specimen collection, transportation to the laboratory, analysis turnaround time; result disclosure to families, (iii) counselling to families; and, (iv) referral to treatment clinic. A number of key themes from this 'Getting To Outcomes' (10 steps) assessment process require urgent implementation by Kaduna State through the setting up of steering committee to address the issues that were raised regarding the Objectives of a SCD programme, Perceptions, and Implementation of NBS. For the State to adopt Community based approach by involving Volunteer Community Mobilisers (VCMs) and Traditional Birth Attendants (TBAs) for maximum benefit and to ensure that a robust monitoring and evaluation process is in place.

Author Contributions: Conceptualization, K.A.A., L.H., A.L., B.P.D.I. and B.O.; Methodology, K.A.A., L.H., A.L., B.P.D I. and B.O.; Formal Analysis, L.G., E.G. and K.A.A.; Resources, B.P.D., L.G.D. and I.I.; Data Curation, L.G., E.G., K.A.A. and B.O.; Writing-Original Draft Preparation, K.A.A., B.P.D.I, L.H., A.L., L.G.D., B.O., I.I., W.A.; Writing-Review & Editing, B.P.DI., K.A.A., L.H., A.L., L.G.D., B.O., I.I., W.A.

Funding: This research received no external funding.

Acknowledgments: We are sincerely indebted to the invaluable leadership and support of Paul Dogo, Commissioner of Health—Kaduna State, regarding the development and implementation of Newborn Screening in Kaduna State. We acknowledge Amina Abubakar Bello, wife of Niger state Governor for facilitating her state's involvement in the Focus group activity in Kaduna. We are very grateful to all the participants of the two day focus group workshops, and Barau Dikko Teaching Hospital, Kaduna.

Conflicts of Interest: The authors declare no conflict of interest

References

1. Secretariat FNWHA. Sickle Cell Anaemia. 2006. Available online: http://apps.who.int/gb/ebwha/pdf_files/WHA59-REC3/WHA59_REC3-en.pdf (accessed on 30 August 2018).
2. Williams, T.N. Sickle Cell Disease in Sub-Saharan Africa. *Hematol. Oncol. Clin. N. Am.* **2016**, *30*, 343–358. [CrossRef] [PubMed]
3. World Health Organisation. Sickle-Cell Anaemia Report by the Secretariat. Fifty Ninth World Health Assembly 2006. Available online: http://apps.who.int/gb/ebwha/pdf_files/WHA59/A59_9-en.pdf (accessed on 30 August 2018).
4. Piel, F.B.; Patil, A.P.; Howes, R.E.; Nyangiri, O.A.; Gething, P.W.; Dewi, M.; Temperley, W.H.; Williams, T.N.; Weatherall, D.J.; Hay, S.I. Global epidemiology of Sickle haemoglobin in neonates: A contemporary geostatistical model-based map and population estimates. *Lancet* **2013**, *381*, 142–151. [CrossRef]
5. Inusa, B.P.; Juliana Olufunke, Y.D.; John Dada, L. Sickle Cell Disease Screening in Northern Nigeria: The Co-Existence of Thalassemia Inheritance. *Pediatr. Ther.* **2015**, *5*, 3–6. [CrossRef]
6. Makani, J.; Cox, S.E.; Soka, D.; Komba, A.N.; Oruo, J.; Mwamtemi, H.; Magesa, P.; Rwezaula, S.; Meda, E.; Mgaya, J.; et al. Mortality in sickle cell anemia in Africa: A prospective cohort study in Tanzania. *PLoS ONE* **2012**, *6*, e14699. [CrossRef] [PubMed]
7. Eccles, M.P.; Mittman, B.S. Welcome to implementation science. *Implement. Sci.* **2006**. [CrossRef]
8. Anie, K.A.; Treadwell, M.J.; Grant, A.M.; Dennis-Aantwi, J.A.; Asafo, M.K.; Lamptey, M.E.; Ojodu, J.; Yusuf, C.; Otaigbe, A.; Ohene-Frempong, K. Community engagement to inform the development of a sickle cell counselor training and certification program in Ghana. *J. Community Genet.* **2016**, *7*, 195–202. [CrossRef] [PubMed]
9. Swainston, K.; Summerbell, C. *The Effectiveness of Community Engagement Approaches and Methods for Health Promotion Interventions*; University of Teeside: Teeside, UK, 2008.
10. CDI Study Group. Community-directed interventions for priority health problems in Africa: Results of a multicountry study. *Bull. World Health Organ.* **2010**, *88*, 509–518. [CrossRef] [PubMed]
11. Chinman, M.; Hunter, S.B.; Ebener, P.; Paddock, S.M.; Stillman, L.; Imm, P.; Wandersman, A. The getting to outcomes demonstration and evaluation: An illustration of the prevention support system. *Am. J. Community Psychol.* **2008**, *41*, 206–224. [CrossRef] [PubMed]

12. Meyers, D.C.; Durlak, J.A.; Wandersman, A. The quality implementation framework: A synthesis of critical steps in the implementation process. *Am. J. Community Psychol.* **2012**, *50*, 462–480. [CrossRef] [PubMed]
13. Wandersman, A.; Alia, K.; Cook, B.S.; Hsu, L.L.; Ramaswamy, R. Evidence-Based interventions Are Necessary but Not Sufficient for Achieving Outcomes in Each Setting in a Complex World: Empowerment Evaluation, Getting to Outcomes, and Demonstrating Accountability. *Am. J. Eval.* **2016**, *37*, 544–561. [CrossRef]

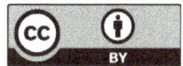
© 2018 by the authors. Licensee MDPI, Basel, Switzerland. This article is an open access article distributed under the terms and conditions of the Creative Commons Attribution (CC BY) license (http://creativecommons.org/licenses/by/4.0/).

MDPI
St. Alban-Anlage 66
4052 Basel
Switzerland
Tel. +41 61 683 77 34
Fax +41 61 302 89 18
www.mdpi.com

International Journal of Neonatal Screening Editorial Office
E-mail: ijns@mdpi.com
www.mdpi.com/journal/ijns

www.ingramcontent.com/pod-product-compliance
Lightning Source LLC
LaVergne TN
LVHW071954080526
838202LV00064B/6746